HEALTHY START

A PEDIATRICIAN'S PRESCRIPTION FOR HEALTHY BABIES & HAPPY MOTHERS

Author

Dr. Imran Patel

Published By

Invincible Publication Pvt. Ltd.

Published by:

Invincible Publication Pvt.Ltd.

201A, SAS Tower, Sector 38, Gurugram, Haryana – 122003

Website : www.invinciblepublishers.com

Sales Office : - 4760-61/23, Basement, Pratap Street, Ansari Road,

Daryaganj, New Delhi - 110002

Email: invinciblepublishers@gmail.com

ISBN : 978-93-58863-92-5

Book Name : Healthy Start: A Pediatrician's prescription for healthy babies & happy mothers

Author: Dr. Imran Patel

Developmental Editor- Raveena Paul

First Edition: 2024

DISCLAIMER

This book is written to provide general guidelines and raise awareness about pregnancy, childbirth, and early childhood development. The information presented here is based on my experience and knowledge as an MD in pediatrics. However, it is important to understand that each individual case is unique, and the recommendations provided in this book may not be suitable for every situation.

While I strive to offer accurate and up-to-date information, this book is not a substitute for professional medical advice, diagnosis, or treatment. Always seek the advice of your physician, pediatrician, or other qualified healthcare provider with any questions you may have regarding a medical condition or before making any changes to your health regimen. Never disregard professional medical advice or delay in seeking it because of something you have read in this book.

The author and publisher disclaim any liability or responsibility for any loss, injury, or damage incurred as a consequence, directly or indirectly, of the use or application of any of the contents of this book. The reader should consult their healthcare provider to determine the appropriateness of the information for their specific situation.

This book is intended to complement, not replace, the relationship between a patient and their own medical provider. The guidance provided here is meant to support and inform, not to replace the personalized care and professional judgment of your healthcare team.

By using this book, you acknowledge and agree that you have read and understand this disclaimer and that you take full responsibility for your health decisions and actions.

ABOUT THE BOOK

As an MD in pediatrics, Dr. Imran Patel has witnessed firsthand the challenges parents face in today's world. He understands that navigating the complexities of childcare can feel like finding your way through a maze without a map. This book is specifically crafted to empower mothers—whether they are planning to have a child, currently with a child, or have recently become parents—to navigate this life-changing journey with knowledge and confidence.

The book aims to provide a pediatrician's prescription in its simplest form, offering comprehensive answers to all your parenting questions in one accessible resource. By bridging the gap between accurate medical information and modern parenting needs, it seeks to simplify the process and cast away the anxieties caused by advice coming in from all directions.

ACKNOWLEDGEMENT

First and foremost, I extend my heartfelt thanks to the countless mothers, fathers, and caregivers whose insights, experiences, and traditions have shaped the content of this book. Your wisdom and willingness to share have enriched this work immeasurably.

I am indebted to my mentors, my team and partners at Asian Children Hospital, to medical professionals and researchers at large, whose tireless efforts continue to advance our understanding on infant care and postnatal practices.

I would like to express my appreciation to Invincible's publishing team and my editor, Raveena Paul for their guidance and support throughout the writing process. Your expertise and commitment have helped refine this book into its final form.

Lastly, I extend my gratitude to my family, friends, and colleagues for their unwavering encouragement and belief in this project. Your love and support has been a constant source of inspiration for me.

Finally, to my patients and their families, and all those who have followed my journey on social media and beyond, your support and encouragement have been beyond my wildest expectations.

This book is a culmination of my experiences, lessons learned, and the collective wisdom of those who have touched my life. It is my hope that it serves as a guiding light for young parents navigating the complexities of parenthood and pediatric care.

PREFACE

Dr. Imran's Story And Patients' Stories

I was born on 5th August 1988, at a small place near Somnath temple in Gujarat, called Veraval. Carrying dreams and aspirations my parents, Mr. Suleman and Mrs. Zubeda Patel, had shifted from our native place in Mangrol to Veraval. My father used to work as a mining supervisor in a soda ash factory. As a family of 5 people, papa's salary used to be stretched out covering our basic living expenses. Papa had studied in Gujarati medium, and wanted me to get an English-medium education. He believed it would open doors for me that he himself could never access. My mother had studied only up to the 7th standard and somehow she also knew that education was the only way out from the struggle we were in.

We lived in rented houses, moving often from one to another because landlords didn't let us stay for long at one place. My father worked tirelessly, taking extra jobs to support my education. This was contrary to the order of things at our village. Life there was rather simple. The rural life back then did not pay much heed to academics, children were engaged in household chores or playing on the streets. People didn't have much business in pushing their children into academic growth.

My father never wanted me to grow up around that society but he could not do anything about it because of our meager financial resources. However, slowly things started to change, as I was growing up papa had started a side business and few other jobs because of which our financial situation gradually improved and with it my father decided to take control in his hands. Understanding the limitations of our village life, my father made a significant decision. He decided to send me to a boarding school in the city, hoping it would provide the conducive environment needed for my growth. I was in the 8th standard when I left our village and entered a world that demanded discipline and hard work.

Boarding school was a stark contrast to my previous life. We used to wake up at 5 AM and run for 2 kilometers, followed by a strict schedule. The food was different from what I was used to, and the discipline was tough. I often felt homesick, especially on Sundays when we would line up to make phone calls home. Hearing my parents' voices used to make me cry, they would try to console me with their words of encouragement but they knew this was the sacrifice that was meant to be done in order to make something out of my life.

Over time, I adjusted to the boarding school routine. The strict discipline, which had seemed harsh at first, began to instill a sense of responsibility and focus in me. I remembered my father's efforts and my mother's support, which motivated me to work even harder.

I immersed myself in my studies, determined to make my parents proud. The challenges of boarding school were surely immense, however, they slowly transformed me, teaching me the art of taking care of myself, doing my chores, leading a disciplined life and this has been instrumental during my residency days as well.

Scoring well in the 10th standard was a pivotal moment in my life. My father, recognizing my potential, encouraged me to pursue the sciences. His belief in the power of education and his desire for me to have opportunities he never had, drove his decision. I too embraced the path.

It was sometime before that my aspiration to become a doctor had taken their roots. My younger brother, Mohsin, only 4 years old then, was suffering from a serious heart problem. His illness was hard on my family.

My father did not have the money needed for the treatment. Desperate and determined to save his son, he somehow borrowed funds from friends and relatives. And they left for Mumbai, seeking treatment for my brother.

For the month that my brother was in Mumbai undergoing his surgery, my twin sisters Sahida, Jahida and I stayed at our grandmother's place. We were constantly anxious and scared. Every day, we would cry and ask our grandmother, when our brother would come back and if his surgery would be successful. The uncertainty and fear were overwhelming, and those days were some of the hardest we faced as a family.

Seeing my brother go through such a critical surgery and witnessing the emotional and financial toll it took on my family had affected me a lot. It planted a dream of becoming a doctor in me, of someday saving someone's life. I think this is the reason why I wanted to become a doctor and why even today if someone in dire need of medical help comes to me, I just think of saving their life first. I know what families go through when someone they love is not well. I know because I have lived that terror, that uncertainty, and it kills you inside.

Anyways, returning to the course of my life, my brother's ordeal opened my eyes to how deeply illnesses affect families, not just the patients. The stress, fear, and financial strain were immense, but so was the love and support that kept us going. I remember at that time, the doctor who was handling my brother's case was in fact "farishta" to us. We looked up to him to save my brother. And till date I cannot forget this one person whom I have never even met, yet his impact on my life has been immense and everlasting.

This experience solidified my desire to become a doctor. I wanted to help other families facing similar struggles and provide the care and support that my brother received. I wanted to experience the honor and respect regarded to this profession.

The journey from that small village to eventually becoming a pediatrician was driven by these early experiences. My family's challenges and my father's unwavering commitment to our well-being became the foundation for my career choice. It taught me the importance of resilience, compassion, and the profound impact a dedicated doctor can have on a family's life.

After scoring well in the 10th standard, my path became clearer. With my father's support, I gained admission to a prestigious college in Karad Maharashtra for my MBBS(Bachelor of Medicine and Bachelor of Surgery). First year in MBBS was hard, it required a lot of adjusting too. A young boy from a small town needed to test waters in this big state, amongst thousands of students, a fierce battlefield and a dream to stand tall in the crowd of these new faces. I used to struggle with my first-year subjects, and I remember during my finals, I asked the person sitting next to me for help with some questions, but he denied straight to my face. Fast forward a few years to the medicine final, and the same friend went blank and sought my help. This taught me that life has its own way of turning the tables, and you never know how people can be of help to you. I passed my MBBS and I was surprised to see that even after 5.5 years of it, I didn't come out hating the experience (Haha). After MBBS, I felt it in me that I needed more of it, so like most doctors, I too joined the race to become an MD(Doctor of Medicine). I too began working hard. Initially, my dream was of specializing in Orthopaedics. However, when I couldn't secure a seat in that specialty, I had to choose between MD in Medicine or Pediatrics. My fondness for children led me to choose Pediatrics, setting the foundation for my future career as a pediatrician. I started my MD in Mumbai, where I spent the next 3 years studying pediatrics and child healthcare.

During my MD, I was not very fond of the highly competitive environment that existed in the Indian medical sphere. And due to this I wanted to move to Dubai, attracted by the promise of a higher standard of living and better work environment. But my PG guide and my mentor, Dr. V. Kotrashetti sir, who has played an immense role in my journey of becoming a pediatrician, asked me to reconsider my plans. He told me in these exact words, "tu india ke liye bana hai" aur "tu yahi kuch bada karke dikhayega, forget about Dubai and do something worthwhile with your knowledge in this country". I was bound to listen to him, since he was the one that I respected and honored the most (and I hold the same respect and honor for him till date). so somehow I chose to stay in India and let destiny play its role. Looking back now I think that my destiny had laid its course way before I even could figure it out.

I don't think it was by chance that I chose pediatrics, that I did not get a seat in orthopedics, I think it happened exactly how it was meant to be.

After MD, I was trying to carve out a path for myself. The struggle was real, amidst the competitive field of medicine, finding a stable ground was not quite easy. Staying in Mumbai was a little out of my bounds, rent alone would have taken my entire salary if I chose to work there or practice in Mumbai. So, I came to Ahmedabad, where my family had a home and I chose to start my job hunt here. It was during this time that I got a temporary position of a consultant with a trust hospital. However, during my tenure here, I couldn't find satisfaction at the workplace, there was not much tending to patients here as well and I knew that I wanted to do more for people who needed help.

To my benefit, after three months of working there, I was offered an Assistant professor's position at Government Medical College in Ahmedabad. Followed by this I was offered a part-time job at a private hospital. Here, I was able to find good footing and appreciation for my work. My dedication impressed the hospital administration, and they soon offered me a permanent position at their hospital. Eventually, I even established myself as a working partner. This opportunity allowed me to settle at Ahmedabad and focus on my career.

The kind of exposure this trajectory had given me helped me to grow a lot in my career and I wanted to take things further with the idea of one day opening up my own hospital.

With time, this dream did come true and I established my own hospital along with two partners. One of them, Dr. Deepak Somani, was my senior and he has supported me like a brother through thick and thin. When we decided to open the hospital, Dr. Deepak helped me out in every possible way, standing in support always. My second partner, Dr. Hardik Chaudhari, is a doctor of great repute and it has been an amazing experience to witness the kind of work he does on the field. With my team, Asian Children Hospital took its shape and today it is running successfully in Ahmedabad, Gujarat.

Our hospital helped me with professional growth and it not only brought me respect and honor but also allowed me to make a significant impact on the lives of my patients and their families.

In 2017, I got married to my wonderful wife, Dr. Irum Patel, who is a dentist by profession, and together we have been blessed with two amazing children, Haider and Hamdan. Balancing my professional and personal life has been challenging, but also incredibly fulfilling. My wife's understanding and support have been invaluable, allowing me to pursue my career while being an active part of our family life.

It was a few years after this that my journey took another turn. People poured in their love through social media, sharing videos of my interactions with children visiting me for consultations. These videos till date are just simple, unedited cuts from my everyday work, there is nothing extravagant about them, however, the love that people have showered onto me, has been unbelievable and unfathomable.

I just feel happy that I can bring a smile to millions of faces who watch these reels. It has been one of the most unexpected and heartwarming experiences of my life, and I feel blessed each day to have earned such respect and love from people in my country and beyond. Beyond this, I have been told that this social media growth has actually worked to dispel a lot of fears in parents w.r.t topics like vaccination, seeking consultations and have somehow encouraged parents to seek medical guidance. Not only that, this has also initiated a shift in the perception of a doctor's persona, attracting interest from foreign medical institutions into understanding this new vision that we are bringing to the table w.r.t doctors in child healthcare.

What more could I have asked for?

My journey from a small village to becoming a pediatrician was marked by hard work, determination, and the unwavering support of my patients, their families, my own family, and my mentors. Little children who visit my hospital, sometimes in critical conditions, bring joy and relief when they are healed and treated. Their parents often send blessings my way, and I believe it is their blessings that have made it possible for me to reach where I am today. There have been challenges, for sure, but with so much love and support, these challenges only strengthened my resolve to make a difference.

Even through this book, I wish to pass down knowledge to the coming generations who often feel lost and confused during their journeys with their children and their healthcare.

CONTENTS

Chapter 1

THE CULPRIT CULTURE

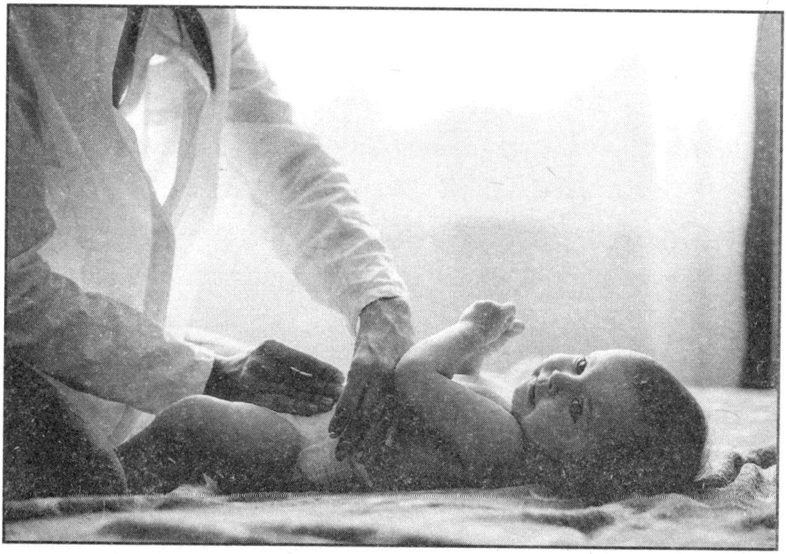

As an MD in pediatrics, I've witnessed firsthand the challenges that parents face in today's world, where navigating the complexities of childcare can feel like finding your way through a maze without a map.

Parenting has become increasingly demanding, with expectations weighing heavily on the shoulders of young moms and dads. There is too much confusion as to what is right for your babies, that parents find themselves torn apart between multitude of advice and suggestions. In addition to this, there is a growing market, exploiting this confusion around parenting and childcare, blindly pushing their products and services onto these parents.

I refer to this phenomenon as the "culprit culture," which is the result of various factors that have made parenting more complex than ever before. From the relentless pressure to raise high-achieving children to the overwhelming influx of information from digital sources, and marketed products projecting the never ending choices, parents are bombarded with stress from all directions.

In the midst of this overload, it's no wonder that parents find themselves feeling confused and uncertain about even the smallest aspects of childcare. They grapple with questions about sleep routines, diseases, discipline strategies, child cues, nutrition and more, all while striving to provide the best possible care for their children.

The culprit culture encompasses a multitude of influences, including societal norms, cultural expectations, technological advancements, marketing and shifting family dynamics. It perpetuates the belief that there is a "perfect" way to parent and places unrealistic standards on parents to meet these ideals.

As a pediatrician, I strive to support parents in navigating this complex landscape by providing evidence-based guidance, practical advice, and reassurance that "You can do it". I encourage parents to trust their instincts, prioritize their child's well-being, and filter out the excess overload that is out there.

Mother Knows Best

Look at the irony of our human existence. We trust everything else but the source where we came from. Human body is made up of the elements found in nature. She created us, she nurtured us and gave us everything that we needed in order to survive. I always say "God is kind", "Nature is kind". Before a woman became a mother, she too was in the lap of the greatest mother of all, mother nature, nourished by her, nurtured by her, cared for by her. Mother nature knows what's best, she knows the 'what, when and how'. Nature created the very essence of human existence. You don't have to know how things work and yet your body works exactly how it should.

Evolution took millions of years to form our bodies, our minds, and their intelligence is far beyond what we can consciously know of. We do not give much credit to the body's innate intelligence. With each obstacle, each problem, each infection your body learns to fight better, to hold resilience and to adapt, to ensure your survival. You have an intelligence inherited in the form of genetics that signals your body to create, to develop and eradicate. Your body knows existence better than you can ever know.

And this is why I say "God is kind", "Mother nature is kind". Everything has been taken care of. It is when we choose to disrespect these systems that we face the wrath of nature.

Just think of this, before a child is born, the womb is prepared in a way, where temperatures, fluids, nourishment everything is set to the levels which makes it possible to create and protect the new life. When a child is born, the milk is supplied with each nutrient that is necessary for the baby's development. Its formulation is just perfect. It is made in a way that ensures that the food is easy to digest for a living being that has just entered earth, one that doesn't know the meaning of food, hunger, fulfillment, yet nature takes care of it through the mother's body.

From the moment of conception, the mother's body undergoes a series of remarkable changes to support the developing fetus.

During pregnancy, the mother's body experiences a surge of hormones that initiate a cascade of physiological adaptations. The uterus expands to accommodate the growing baby, while the placenta forms to provide essential nutrients and oxygen. The mother's blood volume increases, her heart works harder, and her metabolism shifts to meet the demands of pregnancy.

As the baby grows, the mother's body continues to adapt. Her breasts enlarge and produce milk to nourish the newborn after birth. Meanwhile, her joints loosen to prepare for childbirth, and her pelvic floor muscles stretch to accommodate the baby's passage through the birth canal.

After childbirth, the mother's body undergoes further changes as it begins the process of recovery and healing. Hormonal shifts trigger the release of milk for breastfeeding, while the uterus contracts to its pre-pregnancy size.

Since the beginning of human civilization, the mother's body was where everything began. Our traditional systems had extensive knowledge of the aspects of pregnancy, conception, delivery and child care. But with time, some gaps emerged in these systems.

The culprit culture made us forget about one very important aspect to childcare and this is the innate wisdom that is present within us. We are left to feel lost, where companies know better, they know better what food your baby wants, what drinks, formula, and substitutes are best for our children. And young mothers are made to feel they know nothing.

Nature provided a woman with what we call as the mother's instincts, a powerful force that should never be underestimated. It's a result of millions of years of evolution and is passed down through generations.

During pregnancy, a mother's instincts kick in, guiding her in making choices that promote the health and safety of her unborn baby. And when the baby is born, a mother's intuition continues to play a vital role in her parenting journey. From deciphering her baby's cries to knowing when something isn't quite right, a mother's instincts are always at work, helping her navigate the ups and downs of motherhood.

As a doctor, I believe that if nature trusts a mother's body and mind for her progeny, why shouldn't humans believe in it too. Whatever mechanisms your body develops during this time, it biologically makes it possible to say that for a child, "The mother knows best" and you should believe in it too. Start your journey with this faith that Nature has given me everything to navigate this change in my life and to take care of my baby in the best way.

Chapter 2

A GUIDE FOR EXPECTING MOTHERS

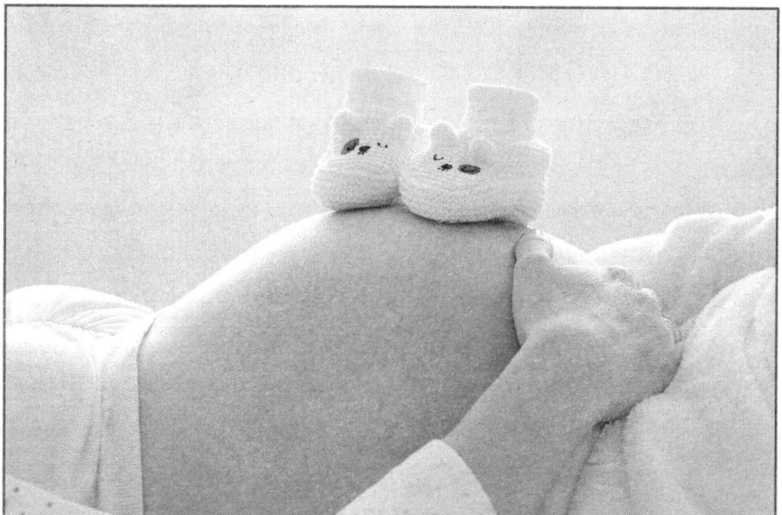

When a woman first discovers she is pregnant, it's a really confusing moment, for some it brings immense joy, for some it is a daunting moment representing the changes that are about to happen, but I think it's not always one emotion, it's a mix of a lot. She may have been dreaming of this moment for years or it might have happened all of a sudden. Every expecting mother begins her journey with the question, "Am I really ready for this?"

See, preparation can only be made easy by gaining knowledge on the subject. Your best bet is by knowing the things and the changes that are about to happen in your body. Don't rely on others to know what is going to happen in the next months, invest your time and energy in being the one who is most prepared and most knowledgeable on the know how.

So, I am going to first explain as to what actually happens in the body when a woman conceives, and we will travel together through the entire journey of being pregnant. When you know your body inside out, it becomes easy to accept the changes that you will be going through.

Pregnancy involves all three aspects of your existence, body, mind and psyche. There will be changes that will happen in all these three aspects and knowing about the science behind them, helps to soften the blow.

Firstly, your body will change in every aspect, your mind will undergo changes on the basis of hormonal fluctuations that will happen inside, and these changes will further lead to emotional states that will affect your psyche.

See our body has a chemical system running inside us, these chemicals are called hormones. Most of our vital organs are assigned a particular hormone to it, and these hormones signal how our body should be and based on that how our emotions and feelings should occur. All the hormones in the body answer to the master gland called as pituitary, which regulates their release. During pregnancy a female's hormones go through a swinging change, there are some hormones that take the driver seat and help the woman to prepare her body and mind for the baby that is going to live inside of you. When these hormones rise in levels, it creates certain effects, like morning sickness, mood swings, fatigue etc.

Now let's start from the beginning how these changes take place.

Conception

Our story begins with an egg and a sperm meeting in the fallopian tube. The moment the sperm penetrates the egg, magic happens. This single cell, called a zygote, is where your baby's life starts.

First Month: The Early Days (Weeks 1-4)

The zygote begins its journey to the uterus, dividing and multiplying into a cluster of cells known as a blastocyst. Around day five or six, the blastocyst implants itself into the rich lining of the uterus. This marks the official start of pregnancy.

In the early weeks, emotions are a whirlwind. One moment you will feel elated, imagining the future with your baby; the next, you find yourself crying over small things. Morning sickness strikes hard during this time, causing tiredness and fatigue. This time period requires a little bit of adjusting to.

Hormones At Play:

- **hCG** (human chorionic gonadotropin) is released, which

supports the pregnancy and signals the body to stop menstruation.

- **Mental Health:** This early stage may bring subtle changes in mood and feelings, often mixed with excitement and anxiety about the new life growing within.

Second Month: Setting The Stage (Weeks 5-8)

The cells rapidly divide and begin to specialize. The tiny heart starts beating around week six, a major milestone. Major organs like the brain, spinal cord, and kidneys start to form.

Hormones At Play:

- **Oestrogen and Progesterone** levels rise to support the growing embryo.
- **Physical Changes:** Morning sickness, fatigue, and breast tenderness are common due to these hormonal surges.
- **Mental Health:** Mood swings and emotional variability can occur as the body adjusts to these changes.

Third Month: The Fetus Takes Shape (Weeks 9-12)

Now called a fetus, the developing baby continues to grow. By the end of this month, the fetus has developed vital organs, and the tiny heart is beating steadily.

Hormones At Play:

- **hCG** levels peak and then stabilize, often reducing the severity of morning sickness.
- **Physical Changes:** The uterus expands, and the mother might start showing a small baby bump.
- **Mental Health:** The risk of miscarriage drops, often

reducing anxiety. However, the anticipation and emotional adjustments continue.

Second Trimester: Growth And Development (Months 4-6)

Fourth Month: Rapid Growth (Weeks 13-16)

The fetus grows rapidly, developing more distinct facial features and limbs. The placenta is now fully developed, taking over hormone production.

Hormones At Play:

- **Placental Hormones** stabilize the pregnancy.
- **Physical Changes:** Increased energy levels and a decrease in morning sickness. The baby bump becomes more noticeable.
- **Mental Health:** Many women feel a renewed sense of energy and well-being. Excitement builds as they start to feel fetal movements, known as "quickening."

Fifth Month: Building Connections (Weeks 17-20)

The fetus's sensory development is underway. It can hear sounds and may respond to the mother's voice. The body grows, and fine hair called lanugo covers its skin.

Hormones At Play:

- **Steady Hormone Levels** support ongoing growth.
- **Physical Changes:** Continued weight gain, back pain, and heartburn are common.
- **Mental Health:** Emotional attachment deepens as the mother feels more frequent movements. Some women may experience fluctuating emotions due to physical discomfort.

Sixth Month: Sensory Development (Weeks 21-24)

The fetus's senses sharpen. It can hear, taste, and touch. The brain and lungs continue to mature, and the fetus gains more fat.

Hormones At Play:

- **Consistent Hormonal Support** from the placenta.
- **Physical Changes:** Noticeable baby movements, leg cramps, and Braxton Hicks contractions (practice contractions) may occur.
- **Mental Health:** Anticipation and connection grow stronger. The mother may start preparing emotionally and practically for the baby's arrival.

Third Trimester: Final Preparations (Months 7-9)

Seventh Month: Maturing Systems (Weeks 25-28)

The fetus's lungs are maturing, preparing for life outside the womb. The brain develops rapidly, and the fetus starts to open its eyes.

Hormones At Play:

- **Hormones Supporting Growth** continue to work.
- **Physical Changes:** Increased fetal movements and growth spurts. Shortness of breath and difficulty sleeping are common.
- **Mental Health:** Many women experience a mix of excitement and anxiety as the due date approaches.

Eighth Month: Gaining Strength (Weeks 29-32)

The fetus continues to gain weight and build fat stores. The brain's development accelerates, and the baby starts to practice breathing movements.

Hormones At Play:

- **Hormones Maintain Pregnancy** and prepare the body for labor.
- **Physical Changes:** More pronounced back pain, pelvic pressure, and frequent urination.
- **Mental Health:** Increased impatience and readiness for the baby's arrival. Emotional support from family and friends becomes crucial.

Ninth Month: Ready For Birth (Weeks 33-36)

The fetus moves into a head-down position, preparing for birth. The lungs are nearly fully developed, and the baby continues to gain weight.

As the due date approaches, your emotions can intensify. You might feel a mix of excitement and nervousness. The physical discomforts of the third trimester—back pain, swollen feet, and sleepless nights—test your patience

Hormones At Play:

- **Oxytocin** levels rise, preparing for labor contractions.
- **Physical Changes:** The cervix begins to dilate and efface (thin out) in preparation for birth. The baby is fully developed and ready for birth.
- **Mental Health:** Excitement and anxiety peak. Many women experience a nesting instinct, preparing their home for the baby.

How Are These Changes Going To Affect You?

Mood Swings

- **Impact:** The surge of hormones such as estrogen and progesterone plays a significant role in regulating mood. These hormonal fluctuations can cause sudden and unpredictable changes in emotions.
- **Experience:** You might find yourself experiencing intense happiness one moment and irritability or sadness the next. Small triggers, such as a touching commercial or a minor inconvenience, can evoke strong emotional responses.
- **Management:** Recognizing that mood swings are a normal part of pregnancy can help in managing them. Engaging in relaxation techniques, maintaining a balanced diet, and getting enough rest are crucial in stabilizing mood.

Anxiety And Stress

- **Impact:** Pregnancy often brings about concerns regarding the baby's health, the process of labor and delivery, and the impending lifestyle and relationship changes.
- **Experience:** These concerns can lead to heightened anxiety and stress levels. Common worries include whether the baby will be healthy, how to manage the pain of childbirth, and how to balance new responsibilities.
- **Management:** Talking about these concerns with a healthcare provider, attending prenatal classes, and staying informed about what to expect can reduce anxiety. Practicing mindfulness and seeking support from loved ones also helps in managing stress.

Depression

- **Impact:** Some women may experience prenatal depression, which goes beyond the usual mood swings and anxiety. This condition is characterized by persistent feelings of sadness, a lack of interest in daily activities, and feelings of hopelessness.
- **Experience:** Symptoms may include trouble sleeping, changes in appetite, fatigue, and difficulty concentrating. Women with a history of depression or those experiencing significant life stressors are more at risk.
- **Management:** It's important to seek professional help if you experience symptoms of depression. Therapists can provide support through counseling or therapy, and in some cases, medication may be necessary. Support from family and friends, as well as self-care practices, can also play a critical role in managing depression.

Changes In Self Perception, Body Image And Identity

During pregnancy, a woman's body also undergoes dramatic changes, including weight gain, skin changes, and the development of stretch marks. These transformations are essential for supporting the growing baby but can impact how a woman feels about her body.

Hormones like estrogen and progesterone, which rise significantly during pregnancy, contribute to changes in body shape and size. These hormones can also affect skin elasticity and fat distribution. The increase in body size and weight is due to the growing uterus, amniotic fluid, placenta, and the baby itself. Hormonal changes can lead to water retention, contributing to swelling in different body parts. Estrogen and progesterone can also affect skin pigmentation, leading to conditions like melasma (dark patches on the skin). These physical changes can affect a woman's self-esteem and body image. Society's ideals and personal expectations of physical appearance can exacerbate these feelings, leading to anxiety or discomfort about one's changing body.

Becoming a mother involves a significant shift in identity. This transition can bring immense joy and fulfillment but also anxiety and uncertainty as women adjust to their new role. The anticipation of the responsibilities of motherhood, such as caring for a newborn and balancing different aspects of life, can be overwhelming.

The brain undergoes changes during pregnancy and postpartum, with increased activity in areas related to empathy, anxiety, and social interaction. These changes are thought to help mothers bond with their babies and be more attuned to their needs. This heightened sensitivity can also make women more susceptible to anxiety and stress as they adapt to their new role.

The expectations of motherhood, both self-imposed and societal, can contribute to feelings of inadequacy or pressure. Pregnancy can also alter relationships with partners, family members, and friends. The anticipation of a new baby brings about a shift in priorities and dynamics within these relationships. The physical and emotional demands of pregnancy can lead to increased dependency on partners and family for support. The hormone oxytocin, which increases during pregnancy, plays a key role in bonding and social relationships. While it promotes bonding and intimacy, it can also heighten the need for emotional support and closeness from loved ones.

These changes can lead to greater intimacy and strengthened bonds, but they can also cause tension if expectations and needs are not communicated effectively. Partners might feel the stress of impending parenthood differently, leading to misunderstandings or conflicts that require open communication and adaptability.

Now you know the 'why' behind your changing body, mind and psyche. You know why things happen or are happening the way they are. Next big step is to navigate through these changes efficiently.

Psychology

We do not really care for our brain a lot. It is a common misconception that the adult brain cannot change and that they are fixed in patterns. People take pride in living through this rigidity of psychology and behavioral patterns. However, your brain has an ability to change, which is called neuroplasticity. And dawning on a responsibility to cater to the new life, you should take extra care as to how your psyche is functioning around this new YOU.

In India, the complications around pregnancy are often discarded as something that every woman goes through and that it shouldn't be a "BIG DEAL" for you. Afterall, everyone does it, so you are really not that special.

But I always say, it is a big deal. Your particular case is a special one, because there are several factors that make your pregnancy different from others. You are carrying life within you. Your body is nurturing an entire living being inside of you. How can you believe when someone else says, "that it is nothing different, it is what women have been doing for so long and that you should not make a fuss about it"?

This is where the psychology of a woman gets extremely affected. And more often than not this effect is not visible on the surface, it hides beneath layers and shows itself in bits and pieces.

Science and spirituality both say that a child becomes receptive in the womb and a part of its learning happens inside. During this time, it is of utmost importance that a woman takes care of her mental and physical health.

Pregnancy is a significant period involving a multitude of physical, emotional, and psychological changes. Understanding and addressing these psychological aspects is crucial for the well-being of both the mother and the developing baby. Therefore always be mindful about what you are consuming as food for thought for your brain, as your child is "listening".

Your mental state during pregnancy also undergoes changes, as I told you during pregnancy there are hormones that undergo changes in their levels, causing certain emotional fluctuations.

Practical Tips For Psychological Well-Being

1. Understand that it's normal to have a range of emotions and that it's okay to seek help.
2. Having a plan for labor and delivery can provide a sense of control and preparedness.
3. Keep a journal to note positive experiences and milestones throughout the pregnancy.
4. Practices like meditation, deep breathing exercises, and yoga can reduce stress and promote emotional well-being.
5. Regular physical activity, a balanced diet, and adequate sleep are essential for mental health.

6. Maintaining strong connections with family, friends, and partners is crucial for emotional support.

When To Seek Help

If a pregnant woman experiences persistent feelings of sadness, anxiety, or distress that interfere with daily functioning, it is important to seek professional help. Symptoms such as severe mood swings, inability to function in daily life, or thoughts of harming oneself or the baby require immediate attention from a healthcare provider.

Pregnancy is a profound period of change for a woman, encompassing not only physical transformations but also deep emotional and psychological adjustments. As she navigates this journey, she often finds herself letting go of parts of her former self to make space for the new life growing within her. This transition involves embracing a new identity and the myriad responsibilities of impending motherhood. During this critical time, the support of family and, especially, her partner is paramount. Without this support, the challenges can become overwhelming, making an already complex process much more difficult.

The role of the partner is particularly crucial. A supportive partner can provide emotional stability, practical help, and a sense of shared responsibility, all of which are essential for the well-being of the pregnant woman. The presence of a caring partner can alleviate many of the stresses associated with pregnancy, from managing household tasks to providing comfort and reassurance. In contrast, a lack of support or conflict within the relationship can exacerbate feelings of isolation and anxiety.

Family dynamics also play a significant role. Unrealistic

expectations and pressure from family members can lead to increased stress and emotional distress. Cultural and familial expectations about pregnancy, childbirth, and parenting can sometimes be unrealistic or at odds with the woman's own preferences and needs. This pressure can result in heightened cortisol levels, a stress hormone that, when chronically elevated, can have detrimental effects on both the mother and the developing baby.

Stress during pregnancy is not just an emotional burden; it has tangible physiological effects. Chronic stress can lead to hormonal imbalances, particularly in the levels of cortisol and other stress hormones. These hormonal changes can affect the placenta and the blood flow to the fetus, potentially leading to complications such as preterm birth, low birth weight, and developmental issues. The baby's brain development can also be impacted, potentially increasing the risk of emotional and behavioral problems later in life.

To mitigate these risks, it is essential for the pregnant woman to have a strong support system. Open communication with her partner and family about her needs and feelings can help in creating a supportive environment. Additionally, seeking external support, such as professional counseling or joining support groups, can provide the necessary emotional stability and practical advice. This supportive network not only benefits the mother's emotional health but also contributes to a healthier pregnancy outcome.

Nutrition During Pregnancy: Nourishing Both Mother And Baby

Proper nutrition is vital during pregnancy as it supports the health and development of the baby while maintaining the mother's well-being. Understanding what to eat and what to avoid can make a significant difference in pregnancy outcomes.

There are so many suggestions from relatives and the "experts" that it confuses the expecting mother as to what is good for her and her baby and what is not. However, if you simply just learn what nutrients are required during that time, you can match them to the foods you can easily accommodate in your diet. See, humans have been living through centuries, and there are so many practices around the world around food, when it comes to pregnancy and childbirth. You cannot and should not follow all of them. You should just learn about the nutrients that are required by your body during this time and then include them through your diet, or take help from your doctor to chart out ways in which you can fulfill the nutritional requirements.

Key Nutritional Components

1. **Folic Acid (Folate)**- Essential for the development of the neural tube, which develops into the brain and spinal cord.
2. **Iron**- Supports the increased blood volume and prevents anemia, which can cause fatigue and complications during delivery.
3. **Calcium**- Essential for the development of the baby's bones and teeth, and maintaining the mother's bone health.
4. **Protein**- Crucial for the growth of fetal tissues, including the brain, and maternal tissue growth.
5. **Omega-3 Fatty Acids**- Supports the development of the baby's brain and eyes.
6. **Fiber**- Helps prevent constipation, a common issue during pregnancy.

Foods To Avoid

1. High-Mercury Fish

Mercury can harm the developing nervous system of the baby.

- **Examples:** Shark, swordfish, king mackerel, and tilefish.

2. Raw or Undercooked Foods

Risk of bacterial infections (such as listeria or salmonella), which can be harmful to both mother and baby.

- **Examples:** Raw fish (sushi), undercooked meat, and unpasteurized dairy products.

3. Alcohol And Caffeine

Alcohol can cause fetal alcohol spectrum disorders, and high caffeine intake is linked to miscarriage and low birth weight.

- **Guideline:** Avoid alcohol entirely and limit caffeine intake to less than 200 milligrams per day (about one 12-ounce cup of coffee).

Nutrition Guide For Pregnant Women-

Please check with your doctor before starting with any new diet or dietary addition.

First Trimester (Weeks 1-12)

Nutritional Needs

- **Folic Acid:** Essential to prevent neural tube defects.
  - **Sources:** Leafy green vegetables, citrus fruits, beans, fortified cereals.
- **Iron:** Supports increased blood volume and prevents anemia.
  - **Sources:** Spinach, lentils, chickpeas, lean meats.

- **Vitamin B6:** Helps alleviate morning sickness.
  - **Sources:** Bananas, nuts, whole grains, potatoes.
- **Hydration:** Vital for overall health and reducing nausea.

Recommended Foods

- Leafy greens, citrus fruits, whole grains, lean meats, nuts, seeds.
- Small, frequent meals to manage nausea.

Common Myths

- **Myth:** "Eating sour foods causes miscarriage."
  - **Fact:** There is no scientific evidence to support this. Sour foods, like citrus fruits, are rich in vitamins and safe in moderation.

Second Trimester (Weeks 13-26)

Nutritional Needs

- **Calcium and Vitamin D:** Essential for fetal bone development.
  - **Sources:** Dairy products, fortified plant milk, leafy greens, fish.
- **Iron:** Continued importance for blood supply.
  - **Sources:** Red meat, spinach, lentils.
- **Omega-3 Fatty Acids:** Important for fetal brain development.
  - **Sources:** Fish (low in mercury like salmon), flaxseeds, walnuts.
- **Protein:** Increased requirement for fetal growth.
  - **Sources:** Lean meats, beans, tofu, dairy.

Recommended Foods

- Dairy products, fish (low in mercury), legumes, lean meats, eggs, nuts.

Common Myths

- **Myth:** "Eating papaya and pineapple induces labor."
  - **Fact:** Moderate consumption of ripe papaya and pineapple is safe. Unripe papaya contains latex which may be harmful, but ripe fruits are nutritious and beneficial.

Third Trimester (Weeks 27-40)

Nutritional Needs

- **Energy:** Increased caloric intake to support fetal growth.
  - **Sources:** Whole grains, fruits, vegetables, protein-rich foods.
- **Vitamin K:** Important for blood clotting.
  - **Sources:** Leafy greens, broccoli, brussels sprouts.
- **Fiber:** Helps prevent constipation, a common issue in late pregnancy.
  - **Sources:** Whole grains, fruits, vegetables, legumes.

Recommended Foods

- High-fiber foods, lean proteins, a variety of fruits and vegetables, and whole grains.

Common Myths

- **Myth:** "Eating for two."
  - **Fact:** Pregnant women need more nutrients, not necessarily double the calories. In the case of twins you can eat 600 more calories than usual, otherwise 250 more calories than usual is sufficient. Overeating can lead to excessive weight gain and complications.

General Dietary Recommendations

Balanced Diet

- **Include:** Variety of fruits and vegetables, lean proteins, whole grains, dairy or fortified alternatives.

- **Avoid:** Excess caffeine, alcohol, raw or undercooked meats, high-mercury fish.

Hydration

- **Importance:** Adequate water intake is crucial for maintaining amniotic fluid levels and preventing dehydration.

Supplements

- **Prenatal Vitamins:** Ensure they provide sufficient folic acid, iron, calcium, and DHA.

Busting Common Myths in Indian Culture

1. **Myth:** "Ghee increases a baby's complexion."
   - **Fact:** Baby's complexion is determined by genetics, not by maternal diet. While ghee is a good source of fat, it should be consumed in moderation.
2. **Myth:** "Saffron in milk makes babies fair."
   - **Fact:** Saffron has no effect on the baby's complexion. It can be consumed in small amounts for its potential mood-enhancing properties but not for altering skin color.
3. **Myth:** "Avoiding spicy foods prevents heartburn."
   - **Fact:** Heartburn is common in pregnancy due to hormonal changes. Spicy foods can exacerbate it in some women, but it's not a universal trigger.
4. **Myth:** "Eating dates can induce early labor."
   - **Fact:** Eating dates, especially in the last trimester, can actually be beneficial. Studies have shown that dates may help with labor by promoting cervical ripening and reducing the need for induced labor without increasing

the risk of preterm delivery, it also reduces the chances of C-section by 48%. Dates are a good source of energy, antioxidants, fiber, and nutrients like potassium and magnesium.

- 35 weeks onwards if you can have 5-6 dates everyday, it can provide the above mentioned benefits.
- **Caution:** If you have pregnancy induced diabetes, or weight gain related issues, consume dates in moderation and only under medical supervision.

Exercise During Pregnancy: Staying Active For Health And Well-Being

Exercise during pregnancy offers a range of benefits for both mothers and babies, supporting overall health and preparing the body for labor and delivery. It's crucial to approach exercise with consideration for safety and individual health needs.

Benefits of Exercise During Pregnancy: Regular physical activity during pregnancy provides numerous advantages:

1. **Improved Cardiovascular Health:** Enhances heart strength and circulation, reducing swelling and lowering the risk of gestational hypertension.

2. **Weight Management:** Helps manage weight gain and reduces the likelihood of complications like gestational diabetes.

3. **Enhanced Mood and Energy:** Boosts endorphins, improving mood, reducing anxiety and depression, and combating fatigue.

4. **Better Sleep:** Aids in reducing pregnancy-related sleep issues by relieving stress and anxiety.

5. **Easier Labor and Delivery:** Strengthens the body, particularly pelvic floor muscles, potentially leading to shorter, less complicated labor.

By incorporating safe and appropriate exercise routines, pregnant women can maintain their health, support their baby's development, and prepare themselves physically and mentally for childbirth and beyond.

Recommendations:

Always check with your doctor before starting any new activities, as every pregnancy is different. Here's a simple guide to physical activities during pregnancy:

First Trimester (Weeks 1-12)

- Walking, swimming, and prenatal yoga.
- **Tips:** Listen to your body, rest when needed, stay hydrated, and avoid overheating.

Second Trimester (Weeks 13-26)

- Brisk walking, swimming, light strength training, and Kegel exercises.
- **Tips:** Keep exercise moderate, use supportive shoes and gear, and be cautious with balance.

Third Trimester (Weeks 27-40)

- Walking, swimming, prenatal yoga, and Kegel exercises.
- **Tips:** Avoid overexertion, rest if uncomfortable, and practice relaxation and breathing techniques for labor.

Remember, gentle and regular exercise can help you stay healthy and prepare for childbirth.

Safety Tips:

1. **Consult Your Healthcare Provider:** Obtain clearance

before starting or continuing an exercise regimen, especially with any pregnancy complications.

2. **Stay Hydrated:** Drink ample water before, during, and after exercise to prevent dehydration.
3. **Avoid Overheating:** Exercise in cool environments, wear breathable clothing, and avoid hot yoga or exercising in hot weather.
4. **Listen to Your Body:** Avoid high-impact activities or sports with injury risks. Stop if you feel dizzy, short of breath, or experience pain.
5. **Focus on Proper Form:** As pregnancy progresses, maintain correct posture and form to minimize injury risk. Consider prenatal fitness guidance if needed.

Q1: What should I do if I feel too tired to exercise?

A1: It's normal to feel more tired during pregnancy. Gentle activities like walking or prenatal yoga can actually boost your energy levels. However, rest is equally important. Listen to your body and don't push yourself too hard. Even short, regular walks can be beneficial.

Q2: Is it okay to travel during pregnancy?

A2: Travel is usually safe during the second trimester (weeks 13-26), as you're likely past the nausea phase and not yet too close to delivery. Avoid long journeys and ensure you stay hydrated, move around regularly to prevent blood clots, and choose destinations with good medical facilities.

Q3: Can I continue working until my due date?

A3: Many women can work until their due date, provided their pregnancy is uncomplicated. However, it's important to listen to your body. Take breaks, avoid heavy lifting, and ensure you're not on your feet for prolonged periods. If your work is physically demanding or stressful, discuss your situation with your doctor.

Q4: Is it safe to practice yoga during pregnancy?

A4: Absolutely. Prenatal yoga is safe and beneficial for most pregnant women. It helps with flexibility, relaxation, and prepares your body for labor. However, avoid poses that require lying flat on your back after the first trimester and any positions that cause discomfort. Always consult your doctor before starting any new exercise routine.

Cues During Pregnancy: Recognizing The Signs

Pregnancy is a dynamic process with various physical and emotional cues indicating the progress of both mother and baby. Sometimes the confusion around these cues and inadequate information around them create anxiety in new mothers.

Understanding these cues can help expecting mothers recognize normal changes as well as potential issues that may require medical attention.

First Trimester Cues (Weeks 1-12)

- **Morning Sickness:** Nausea and vomiting are common due to increased levels of hormones such as hCG and progesterone. While uncomfortable, these are typically normal symptoms.
- **Fatigue:** Increased progesterone can cause sleepiness and fatigue as the body adjusts to supporting a growing fetus.
- **Breast Changes:** Tenderness, swelling, and darkening of the areolas occur as the body prepares for breastfeeding.
- **Spotting and Cramping:** Light spotting and mild cramping can occur as the embryo implants in the uterus.

However, heavy bleeding or severe cramping should prompt immediate medical consultation.

Second Trimester Cues (Weeks 13-26)

- **Quickening:** Around 18-20 weeks, mothers often feel the first movements of the baby, known as quickening, which can be a reassuring sign of fetal health.
- **Energy Levels:** Many women experience a surge in energy and a decrease in morning sickness as hormone levels stabilize.
- **Physical Changes:** The belly starts to show as the uterus expands, and some women may notice stretch marks and skin changes.
- **Braxton Hicks Contractions:** These mild, irregular contractions prepare the uterus for labor but are typically not painful. Regular or painful contractions should be discussed with a healthcare provider.

Third Trimester Cues (Weeks 27-40)

- **Fetal Movement:** Regular movement is a good sign of a healthy baby. A noticeable decrease in movement should be reported to a healthcare provider.
- **Swelling and Discomfort:** Swelling in the ankles, feet, and hands is common due to increased fluid retention. Severe swelling, especially in the face and hands, may indicate preeclampsia and requires immediate attention.
- **Shortness of Breath:** As the baby grows, the uterus can press against the diaphragm, causing shortness of breath.
- **Nesting Instinct:** Many women experience a strong desire to prepare their home for the baby's arrival, a psychological cue known as the nesting instinct.

Fetal Movements:

How can you know if the movement of the baby is normal or not?

A baby doesn't move 24 hours a day as we do not work all the time. A baby has its own rest and wake cycles. However there is a certain number assigned which shows if the movement is normal or not.

How To Monitor Fetal Movements

Timing:

- **After Major Meals:** Lie down on your left side for an hour after each major meal (breakfast, lunch, and dinner).

Position:

- **Left Side:** Lying on your left side improves blood flow to the baby and can make movements more noticeable.

Method:

- **Hand on Belly:** Place a hand on your belly to feel the movements more clearly.

Counting Movements:

- **Hourly Count:** During the one-hour period after each meal, count the number of times the baby moves. Aim for at least 5 movements in this hour.
- **Daily Count:** Collectively throughout the day, your baby should move around 12-13 times. This includes movements felt during the designated post-meal periods and other times of the day.

What Constitutes A Movement?

Types of Movements: Kicks, rolls, and flutters are all considered movements. Hiccups are usually not counted.

Variability: It's normal for the baby to have quiet periods. Babies, like adults, have sleep cycles and might be less active at times.

When To Seek Medical Advice

Decreased Movements: If you notice a significant decrease in fetal movements or if the baby does not move at least 5 times in an hour after meals or 12-13 times in a day, contact your healthcare provider immediately.

Changes in Pattern: Sudden changes in the pattern of movements should also be discussed with your healthcare provider.

Complications During Pregnancy: Recognizing And Responding

While many pregnancies proceed without significant issues, complications can arise, requiring prompt medical attention to ensure the health and safety of both mother and baby.

Danger Signs During Pregnancy That Should Be Consulted With A Doctor

It is crucial for pregnant women to be aware of warning signs that may indicate complications.

1. Vaginal Bleeding

- **First Trimester:** Light spotting can be normal, but heavy bleeding may indicate a miscarriage or ectopic pregnancy.
- **Second and Third Trimesters:** Any bleeding could signal placental issues such as placenta previa or placental abruption.

2. **Severe Abdominal Pain Or Cramps**
   - Persistent or severe pain can indicate conditions such as preterm labor, placental abruption, or even appendicitis.
3. **Severe Headaches**
   - Intense or persistent headaches, especially when accompanied by visual disturbances, can be a sign of preeclampsia.
4. **Blurred Vision Or Visual Disturbances**
   - These symptoms, particularly when combined with headaches, swelling, or high blood pressure, may indicate preeclampsia.
5. **Severe Swelling**
   - Sudden or severe swelling of the hands, face, or feet can also be a sign of preeclampsia.
6. **Reduced Fetal Movement**
   - A noticeable decrease in the baby's movements after 28 weeks of pregnancy should be reported. Regular monitoring as mentioned previously is crucial.
7. **High Fever**
   - A fever over 100.4°F (38°C) that doesn't respond to treatment could signal an infection that needs medical attention.
8. **Pain Or Burning During Urination**
   - This can indicate a urinary tract infection (UTI), which can lead to more serious complications if untreated.
9. **Persistent Nausea And Vomiting**
   - Severe nausea and vomiting that prevent you from keeping food or fluids down (hyperemesis gravidarum) can lead to dehydration and malnutrition.

10. Shortness Of Breath Or Chest Pain

- Difficulty breathing or chest pain could indicate a serious condition such as a blood clot in the lungs (pulmonary embolism).

11. Leaking Fluid

- Any fluid leakage before 37 weeks can indicate preterm premature rupture of membranes (PPROM). After 37 weeks, it may signal the onset of labor.

12. Signs Of Preterm Labor

- Contractions or cramping before 37 weeks, along with back pain or pelvic pressure, can indicate preterm labor.

13. Severe Itching

- Intense itching, particularly on the hands and feet, could be a sign of cholestasis of pregnancy, a liver condition that affects pregnancy.

14. Dizziness Or Fainting

- Frequent dizziness or fainting spells can be a sign of anemia or other health issues that need to be addressed.

15. Sudden Weight Gain

- Rapid weight gain, especially with swelling, could indicate preeclampsia.

Common Complications

- **Gestational Diabetes:** This condition occurs when a woman develops high blood sugar levels during pregnancy. It can increase the risk of large birth weight, preterm birth, and Type 2 diabetes later in life for both mother and child. Regular screening and management with diet, exercise, and medication are essential.

- **Preeclampsia:** Characterized by high blood pressure and signs of damage to other organ systems, usually the liver and kidneys. Symptoms include severe headaches, vision changes, upper abdominal pain, and swelling. Preeclampsia can be life-threatening and typically requires early delivery.
- **Preterm Labor:** Labor that begins before 37 weeks of pregnancy. Symptoms include regular contractions, lower back pain, and pelvic pressure. Early medical intervention can sometimes delay delivery to allow for further fetal development.
- **Placenta Previa:** A condition where the placenta covers the cervix, which can cause severe bleeding during pregnancy and delivery. This condition often requires a cesarean section to safely deliver the baby.
- **Miscarriage:** The loss of a pregnancy before the 20th week. Signs include heavy bleeding, severe cramping, and passing tissue from the vagina. While miscarriages are common, repeated occurrences warrant further medical investigation.

Less Common But Serious Complications

- **Placental Abruption:** The placenta detaches from the uterus before delivery, causing severe bleeding and depriving the baby of oxygen and nutrients. Symptoms include sudden abdominal pain, back pain, and heavy bleeding.
- **Intrauterine Growth Restriction (IUGR):** A condition where the baby is not growing at the expected rate inside the womb. Regular ultrasounds can monitor growth, and

early delivery may be necessary if growth issues are severe.

- **Ectopic Pregnancy:** A pregnancy where the fertilized egg implants outside the uterus, usually in a fallopian tube. This can cause life-threatening bleeding and requires immediate medical intervention.

Traditions And Superstitions In The Indian Context: Insights From A Medical Perspective

In India, pregnancy and childbirth are deeply intertwined with cultural traditions and beliefs, some of which stem from ancient practices and cultural norms. While many traditions promote social support and community involvement, others may perpetuate superstitions that can potentially impact maternal health and well-being.

Traditional Practices

1. Family Involvement And Support

- **Significance:** In Indian culture, pregnancy is often seen as a family affair rather than an individual journey. Family members, especially elderly women, play a significant role in providing emotional support, sharing wisdom, and participating in rituals that celebrate the upcoming arrival of the baby.
- **Medical Perspective:** Family support can positively impact maternal mental health and reduce stress during pregnancy. It fosters a sense of community and can enhance overall well-being.

2. Health Practices

- **Significance:** Traditional medical practices are thought to be harmless as they come from nature; these include pregnancy care, dietary recommendations, herbal supplements, and massage therapies aimed at promoting maternal health and fetal development.

- **Medical Perspective:** While some traditional practices can complement modern medical care, others may lack scientific validation or pose potential risks when not taken under medical guidance. It's essential for healthcare providers to discuss these practices with patients to ensure safe integration with evidence-based medical treatments.

3. Rituals And Blessings

- **Significance:** Various rituals and ceremonies are performed during pregnancy and after childbirth to bless the mother and baby, ward off evil spirits, and promote auspiciousness.
- **Medical Perspective:** Participating in rituals can provide emotional and psychological support to expectant mothers, fostering a sense of cultural identity and connection. However, please ensure that rituals do not compromise medical care or safety.

Superstitions

1. Food Restrictions

- **Belief:** Certain foods, such as spicy or "hot" foods, are believed to cause miscarriage or fetal abnormalities. Conversely, specific foods are considered auspicious and are encouraged during pregnancy.
- **Medical Perspective:** While dietary restrictions based on cultural beliefs may have symbolic significance, there is no scientific evidence linking specific foods to miscarriage or fetal abnormalities. Encouraging a balanced diet that meets nutritional needs is essential.

2. **Taboos And Social Restrictions**
   - **Belief:** Pregnant women are often subjected to various taboos and social restrictions, such as avoiding celebrations, visiting temples, or attending social gatherings, especially during specific phases of pregnancy.
   - **Medical Perspective:** Social restrictions can impact maternal mental health by fostering feelings of isolation or guilt. Healthcare providers should encourage open communication with patients and address concerns while respecting cultural beliefs.

Few Recommended Tests On Pregnancy Timeline:

1. **As Soon As Pregnancy Is Confirmed:**
   - **Dating Scan:** To confirm the due date.
2. **11-14 Weeks:**
   - **Nuchal Translucency (NT) Scan:** To assess the risk of chromosomal abnormalities.
   - **Double Marker Test:** To screen for chromosomal abnormalities.
3. **16 Weeks:**
   - **Quadruple Marker Test:** (Optional, not necessary for every patient) To further screen for chromosomal abnormalities.
4. **20-22 Weeks:**
   - **Anomaly Scan:** To check the baby's anatomy and detect any abnormalities.
5. **32-34 Weeks:**
   - **Interval Growth Scan:** To monitor the baby's growth.
6. **36 Weeks:**
   - **Color Doppler Scan:** To assess the baby's blood flow and placental function.

Blood Tests:

- **Complete Blood Count (CBC):** To check overall health and detect anemia.
- **Blood Group:** To determine the mother's blood type.
- **HIV and HBsAg:** To screen for HIV and Hepatitis B.
- **Random Blood Sugar (RBS):** To check blood sugar levels.
- **Thyroid Profile:** To assess thyroid function.
- **Hemoglobin Electrophoresis:** To detect hemoglobinopathies.
- **Urine Routine:** To check for infections or other conditions.

Additional Care:

- **TT Injection:** Tetanus toxoid injections at the 4th and 5th months of pregnancy.

These tests and scans are crucial for monitoring the health of both the mother and the baby throughout the pregnancy.

Chapter 3

UNDERSTANDING MOTHERHOOD

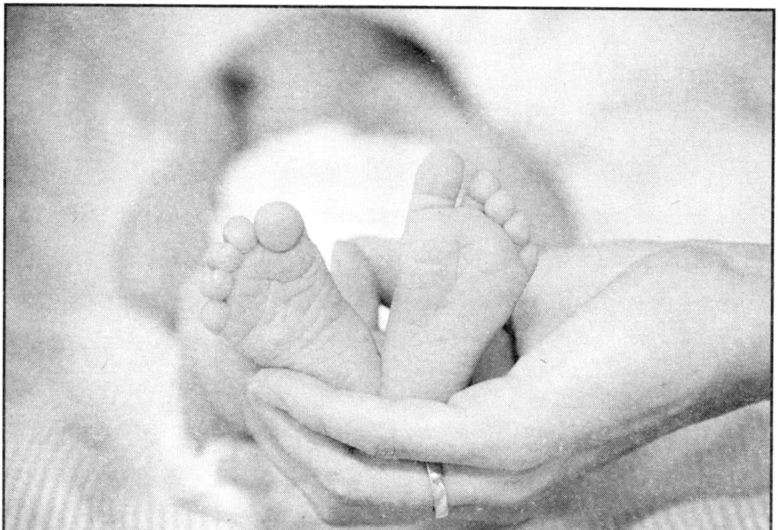

"I've not revealed it to anyone before, but I didn't like her much at first; perhaps because I was really annoyed. I mean, I liked her but not as much as I should. I don't know why (uttering these words in shame)"

"Early after birth, as my baby cried I also used to cry with her. I just wanted to make her sleep. I thought I was unable to do anything and was always concerned that I wouldn't be able to raise her... I found my baby bothersome and felt burdened by her."

"I was alone with my baby, in such a chaotic situation. I found myself wasting a lot of time. I just wandered around at home and couldn't do anything while all the house chores were left undone."

"now I can understand how my mother felt toward me"

Source: Trial Study, NCBI

Sounds Relatable?

Every new mother feels these things after delivering the child.

Things seem to get out of control quickly. Everywhere you see there is chaos and no one seems to be of much help. Most women even find it difficult to understand their baby or even connect with them. Transition to motherhood doesn't happen overnight, as they show in movies, right after a mother holds her baby, she just knows what to do. It doesn't happen like that. Motherhood requires a balance of some skills, some learnings and some emotional development, to reach a stage where you can bond and completely take care of your baby. Every skill is a culmination of practice and without practice how do you expect to become good at something? Women are made to feel that being a mother is all instinctual, you just need to have a baby and you will become a mother.

Well, it's some part instinct and some part practice. So, be patient and know that it's a transition and with practice you will get there.

Transitioning into a mother, every woman goes through three main themes. These themes are named as part of a research that studied new mothers and their behaviors.

Internal Conflicts

In the early postpartum days, mothers often experience conflicting emotions. They may feel unprepared and confused about their new role, thinking it doesn't match their previous expectations. This sense of unpreparedness is heightened by the new expectations they set for themselves and those others have of them.

Many mothers feel inadequate in managing their new responsibilities, losing the sense of control they had before childbirth. This leads to feelings of inconvenience and incapacity, rooted in a lack of confidence. Anxiety about the baby's health and their own feelings toward the child adds to this sense of lost control. New mothers often feel a heightened need for support, reflecting their struggle to adapt.

One mother shared, "Early after birth, as my baby cried I also used to cry with her. I just wanted to make her sleep. I thought I was unable to do anything and was always concerned that I wouldn't be able to raise her... I found my baby bothersome and felt burdened by her."

Some mothers admitted they initially didn't feel the expected maternal affection and felt guilty about it. Another mother confessed, "I've not revealed it to anyone before, but I didn't like her much at first; perhaps because I was really annoyed. I mean, I liked her but not as much as I should. I don't know why (uttering these words in shame)."

Confrontation And Interaction

Over time, the emotional bond between mother and child grows. In the first year, infants' attachment to their mothers is largely based on physical needs like nutrition and protection, which also strengthens the mothers' attachment. Breastfeeding, in particular, fosters a deep connection. Mothers begin to understand that their feelings for their baby go beyond simple love, describing this bond as unlike any other affection they've experienced.

One mother noted, "I feel that it is not just the mother who loves the baby; the baby also develops affection for the mother. When you see that the baby is most comfortable when she finds you close to her and waits to receive your cuddles and hugs you feel, in turn, more attached to her."

Caring for the baby helps mothers learn about their child's characteristics and needs, fostering acceptance and attachment.

Another mother shared, "Since my baby has grown a little bit I feel like he is a grown-up human being sitting beside me; a human being who cannot just speak; I feel that he can understand everything. I talk to him a lot; I think he can understand everything I say. I like him to call me mama as soon as possible. The more I see his reactions, the more I feel affectionate toward him and become more interested in him."

Internalization

As the baby grows, the attachment between mother and child becomes stronger and more enduring. This bond is expressed through a mother's inability to stay away from her child and growing affection. The baby becomes the most important part of the mother's life, and she prioritizes the baby's needs above all else. This deepening attachment helps mothers develop a comprehensive understanding of motherhood, often leading to a newfound appreciation for their own mothers.

Positive Changes

Mothers report positive emotional changes, such as increased compassion, less self-centeredness, and a heightened sense of responsibility. They also experience social growth, becoming more considerate of others, especially children and mothers, and gaining a stronger appreciation for their own parents. Many seek connections with other mothers to discuss child-related topics, showing improved adaptability and flexibility.

Feeling truly grown-up is a sentiment shared by many new mothers, stemming from behavioral changes and a new perspective on life.

Increased attachment to family life and being more thoughtful in decision-making are signs of family stability.

What I am trying to say is that you too will get there someday. The initial months are going to be hard, adjusting to a new life pattern but that's how we learn to adjust right. Our bodies and minds take time to make this new life a part of our old life. But once it does, things appear to be less daunting.

In this chapter I now want to drive your focus to three aspects of recovery w.r.t your body, mind and psyche postpartum.

The Realm Of The Body

What happens to the body after a C-section?

After a C-section, which is a surgical procedure to deliver a baby, the female body undergoes several changes as it recovers. The abdominal muscles, which were cut during surgery, need time to heal. This can cause pain and discomfort, especially when moving or coughing. The incision site itself also needs to heal, and during this time, it's important to keep it clean and dry to prevent infection.

Internally, the uterus, where the baby grew, undergoes a process called involution. This means it gradually shrinks back to its normal size. This process is helped along by breastfeeding, as it triggers the release of hormones that aid in uterine contraction. This contraction helps reduce postpartum bleeding and aids in the recovery of the uterus.

Hormonal changes are also significant after a C-section. Levels of hormones like estrogen and progesterone drop sharply after delivery, which can lead to mood swings and emotional changes. These hormones gradually stabilize over time, but it's common for new mothers to experience ups and downs during this period.

Some women may also experience temporary digestive changes such as bloating, gas, or constipation post-C-section. These issues can be managed with a balanced diet, plenty of fluids, and, if necessary, medications recommended by your healthcare provider.

What happens to the body after vaginal delivery?

After a vaginal delivery, the female body undergoes several changes as it recovers from childbirth. Immediately after giving birth, the uterus begins to contract to expel the placenta and reduce postpartum bleeding. This process, called involution, continues over the next few weeks as the uterus gradually returns to its pre-pregnancy size.

Postpartum bleeding, known as lochia, occurs as the body sheds the uterine lining and excess blood from the birth. This bleeding can last for several weeks, gradually decreasing in amount.

Hormonal changes are significant during this time. Levels of estrogen and progesterone, which were high during pregnancy, drop rapidly after delivery. These changes can lead to mood swings, fatigue, and emotional adjustments as the body adjusts to its new postpartum state.

Physically, the pelvic floor muscles may be weakened or stretched from the delivery process. This can lead to issues like urinary incontinence or discomfort. Gentle exercises and pelvic floor rehabilitation can help strengthen these muscles over time.

Breast changes are also prominent. In response to hormonal shifts, the breasts begin producing colostrum, a nutrient-rich fluid that precedes mature breast milk. Over the first few days after birth, colostrum transitions to milk production as the baby begins breastfeeding or bottle-feeding.

Overall, Postpartum recovery varies from person to person. During this time it is very important for a mother to take her time to heal and rest. It is even more important to follow your healthcare provider's recommendations, w.r.t rest, proper nutrition, and gradually reintroducing physical activity, to support a smooth recovery process.

Complication:

Postpartum Hemorrhage (PPH)

PPH is excessive bleeding after childbirth, defined as blood loss of more than 500ml after a vaginal delivery or 1000 ml after a cesarean section.

PPH can lead to serious complications, including death. It can also lead to problems with recovery, such as anemia and difficulty caring for your baby.

There are a number of factors that can increase your risk of PPH, including low hemoglobin, multiple pregnancy, fibroids,high blood pressure, and a large baby.

Causes:

Tone (Uterine Atony):

- This refers to a poorly contracting uterus after delivery. The muscles fail to clamp down on blood vessels where the placenta was attached, leading to continuous bleeding.
- Weak contractions are the most common cause of PPH, often occurring due to factors like fatigue from a long labor or overdistention of the uterus from multiple babies.

Trauma (Genital Tract Lacerations):

- This refers to tears in the vagina, cervix, or uterus that occur during childbirth. These tears can bleed significantly,especially if they involve larger blood vessels.
- The speaker might discuss how instrumental deliveries (forceps or vacuum) or episiotomy (surgical incision) can increase the risk of trauma-related PPH.

Tissue (Retained Products Of Conception):

- This refers to leftover pieces of placenta or fetal membranes inside the uterus after delivery. These retained tissues can prevent the uterus from contracting properly and continue to bleed.

- The importance of thorough placental examination after delivery can minimize the risk of retained tissue causing PPH.

Thrombin (Coagulopathy):

- This refers to problems with blood clotting. It can be due to pre-existing conditions or complications during delivery that affect the body's ability to form clots and stop bleeding.
- It is really important to check for clotting disorders before delivery and having blood products readily available in case severe PPH occurs due to coagulopathy.
- Recovering from delivery complications
- Postpartum depression & psychology

The best way to prevent PPH is to get regular prenatal care and to follow your doctor's instructions.

If you experience PPH, your doctor will take steps to stop the bleeding and replace any blood that you have lost.

The Realm Of The Mind

Our body works on the interplay of thoughts, hormones, actions and feedback. Our body's chemistry is a highly sophisticated mechanism, however, in its truest essence it is the basis of whatever we feel. Postpartum mood disorders are one of the most highly dreaded topics for new mothers. See, during pregnancy your body had created a surge of certain hormones within you that further produced a certain mood state. When these hormones go back to their old levels, there is a dip in everything you have been feeling.

This is what we call **"Baby blues"**

Baby Blues

The postpartum period can bring a range of emotions for new mothers, with one common experience being the "baby blues." Affecting up to 85% of new moms, this mild, temporary form of depression typically manifests within the first two weeks after giving birth and is characterized by mood swings, anxiety, crying spells, and restlessness.

Causes And Duration

The baby blues are primarily caused by hormonal changes after childbirth. As the body adjusts hormonally, these symptoms usually resolve on their own without medical intervention.

Symptoms

Common Symptoms Include:

- Sudden mood swings
- Anxiety and irritability
- Feeling overwhelmed
- Crying for no apparent reason
- Restlessness

Coping Strategies

- **Rest:** Ensure adequate sleep when possible.
- **Support:** Lean on family and friends for emotional support.
- **Self-care:** Take time for yourself, even if it's just a few moments of relaxation.

In fact, most new moms will experience the baby blues due to hormonal changes. These can cause anxiety, crying, and restlessness but generally subside within two weeks as hormones level out. No mother is happy all the time, and it's normal to feel frustrated or overwhelmed.

Complication

The postpartum period is a time of significant adjustment and recovery. Although pregnancy runs smoothly for most women, in some there may occur certain complications.

Postpartum Depression

One sunny morning, Tanu, a new mother, was cradling her baby and trying to feel the joy she knew she should. Instead, she felt a wave of sadness and fatigue washed over her. These feelings had been persistent since she gave birth a few weeks ago.

Initially, Tanu experienced what she thought were the normal "baby blues," with mood swings, anxiety, and crying spells. However, as the weeks went on, her symptoms intensified. She found it increasingly difficult to bond with her baby and struggled with feelings of worthlessness and guilt. Tanu also noticed changes in her sleep patterns and a significant loss of appetite.

Tanu's history of anxiety during pregnancy and her stressful delivery via emergency cesarean section were significant risk factors. Additionally, the lack of a robust support system and the immense pressure she felt as a new mother contributed to her deteriorating mental health.

One day, her partner noticed her distress and gently suggested that she see a doctor. Reluctantly, Tanu agreed and was diagnosed with postpartum depression (PPD). The doctor explained that PPD is more intense and long-lasting than the baby blues, affecting about 1 in 7 new mothers. It was important to address it promptly to prevent further complications in her ability to function and care for her baby.

Tanu learned that PPD could be influenced by hormonal changes, psychological stressors, and social factors. The doctor emphasized the importance of addressing these areas and encouraged her to start therapy. With her family's support, Tanu began attending therapy sessions and joined a support group for new mothers. She also incorporated mild exercise into her routine and improved her diet, focusing on foods rich in Vitamin B6 to help regulate her mood.

Through therapy, Tanu found her way back to herself. She started to enjoy moments with her baby and felt her anxiety lessened. She realized the significance of seeking help and the strength it took to acknowledge her struggle.

As Tanu you should also know that Postpartum depression is not a matter of shame and you don't need to hide it. If you are going through this or anyone you know is going through this, please seek medical help.

Caring for a newborn is demanding, and with untreated Postpartum depression it can become even more daunting and challenging. During this time be selfish about your mental and physical health and seek care from professionals.

https://www.hopkinsmedicine.org/health/wellness-and-prevention/postpartum-mood-disorders-what-new-moms-need-to-know

https://www.ncbi.nlm.nih.gov/books/NBK304191/

https://www.ncbi.nlm.nih.gov/books/NBK519070/#:~:text=After%20childbirth%2C%20a%20mother%20can,first%202%20weeks%20after%20delivery.

https://www.mayoclinic.org/healthy-lifestyle/labor-and-delivery/in-depth/postpartum-complications/art-20446702

The Realm Of The Society

For a new mother, the major portion of her psychological stress or on the flip side psychological ease comes from the people she is around at that time. If during this time, a mother is pushed into immense emotional stress, her years ahead are gonna be disturbed and affect the way she can care for her child. A mean remark for her, can create scarring for the rest of her life. Sometimes there are remarks making it sound like everything wrong with the baby is all a mother's fault. And she is constantly blamed for getting things right. These things can significantly affect a mother who is still on the edge with all the hormonal and emotional changes happening inside her.

However, if we as a society can learn the right roles, if we can educate our own selves about the process of motherhood, I think we all can be of great help to her.

Traditions And Superstitions

One of the most deeply entrenched parts of the transition to motherhood is the tradition and cultural part.

Every culture has its own set of traditions and superstitions surrounding childbirth and newborn care. While these can provide comfort and a sense of continuity, it's important to balance them with modern medical advice. It's also important to know what is good for the mother and child and what is just blatant shoving down of practices onto the mother. Faith is good but blind faith is disastrous. Parents often find themselves torn between age-old traditions and medical advice.

As a doctor I have witnessed some of these most common practices and I am going to list them down here for you.

Note: I always say that not all traditional practices are good and not all traditional practices are bad, you need to balance and learn to pick and choose the ones that can be scientifically proven to be of benefit.

Good Traditional Practices In Postpartum Care

In India, there are some postpartum related traditional practices that are good at supporting the physical and emotional recovery of mothers.

1. Dietary Guidelines

Traditional postpartum diets in India emphasize nutrition that supports recovery and lactation. Meals typically include easily digestible foods rich in proteins, vitamins, and minerals. Special attention is given to foods believed to aid in healing and milk production. For example, meals may include dishes prepared with seeds and nuts, known for their nutritional benefits. Such dietary practices may be beneficial in promoting the overall well-being of the new mother. However, confirm their safety with a doctor you trust, particularly applying it to your case.

2. Massage And Skin Care

Daily massages using warm oils like sesame or coconut oil are common traditional practices. These massages are believed to aid in muscle relaxation, improve blood circulation, and promote skin hydration. The use of natural oils in massages may serve as therapeutic and nurturing, supporting the mother's physical recovery and emotional well-being.

3. Hygiene And Comfort Measures

Postpartum hygiene practices focus on maintaining cleanliness and comfort for the mother. Warm herbal baths, often prepared with medicinal herbs like neem, are used to cleanse and refresh the body. This practice may promote hygiene and also provides soothing relief to tired muscles.

4. Psychological Support

Cultural practices also prioritize the emotional well-being of new mothers. Supportive environments, avoidance of stress-inducing activities, and encouragement of rest are integral to these traditions. By creating nurturing environments, these practices contribute to the mother's overall psychological well-being during the postpartum period.

5. Modern Adaptations

While rooted in tradition, these practices continue to evolve with modern medical knowledge. Integrating traditional wisdom with evidence-based medical care ensures comprehensive postpartum support for mothers. This approach acknowledges the value of cultural practices while promoting optimal health outcomes through a balanced approach.

Harmful Postpartum Practices In India

Across different regions and cultures in India, several harmful postpartum practices persist despite greater awareness and knowledge. These practices are deeply rooted in age-old traditions, community beliefs, and misconceptions, contributing to potential risks for mothers and newborns. Here are some of the prevalent harmful practices identified:

1. **Personal Care And Hygiene**
    - **Warming Practices and Bathing Restrictions:** In many regions, practices such as immediate bathing of newborns after birth are common. This can lead to hypothermia in newborns due to inadequate temperature regulation.
    - **Poor Hygiene Practices:** Lack of handwashing before and after handling the baby, improper bathing practices, and the use of unsterile cloths or wipes contribute to the risk of infections.

2. **Breastfeeding Practices**
    - **Prelacteal Feeding:** This widespread practice involves giving newborns substances like honey, ghutti, sugar water, or religious water before initiating breastfeeding. Prelacteal feeds delay the initiation of breastfeeding, which is crucial for establishing lactation and providing essential colostrum to the newborn.
    - **Delay in Breastfeeding Initiation:** Many mothers delay breastfeeding initiation due to misconceptions about colostrum (first milk) being harmful or indigestible. Delayed breastfeeding initiation can negatively impact the establishment of breastfeeding and increase the risk of neonatal infections.

3. **Diet and Nutrition Beliefs**
    - **Restrictions on Foods:** Cultural beliefs around "hot foods" e.g. fish, sambhar, rice, jackfruit, papaya, egg) and "cold foods" (e.g. oranges, banana, beans, curd, buttermilk, watermelon, grapes) lead to restrictions that may deprive mothers of nutritious foods necessary for recovery and

lactation. For example, avoiding foods like oranges, bananas, fish, and sambhar can impact maternal nutrition and breast milk quality.

- **Restrictions on Water Consumption:** Some cultures restrict postpartum water consumption under the belief that it can cause prolonged bleeding or abdominal distension. Inadequate hydration can affect maternal health and milk production.

4. Infant/Newborn Care

- **Cord Care Practices:** Applying substances like oil, ghee, turmeric, or herbal mixtures to the newborn's umbilical cord is common but can increase the risk of infections, including neonatal tetanus.
- **Eye Care Practices:** Using unsterile cloths or fingers to wipe the newborn's eyes can introduce pathogens and lead to eye infections.

Myth/Superstition	Explanation
Myth #1: The woman should not drink a lot of water after delivery	Drinking plenty of water is essential for hydration, especially post-delivery when the body needs it for milk production and recovery. Avoiding adequate water intake can lead to dehydration and even the formation of blood clots. This myth is debunked as hydration is crucial for overall health.
Myth #2: Dietary restrictions and preferences	There are numerous myths about what new mothers should and shouldn't eat. While some cultures avoid spicy or pungent foods post-delivery, a balanced diet rich in nutrients supports recovery and lactation. Consuming additional calories from healthy sources like fruits and vegetables is recommended, while moderate intake of ghee can provide essential fats and calories.

Myth #3: More milk consumption improves breastfeeding	While milk is nutritious, excessive consumption doesn't necessarily enhance lactation. Moderation is key, with recommended amounts tailored to individual needs. Overconsumption can lead to issues like lactose intolerance or excess calorie intake.
Myth #4: Breastfeeding should be avoided when sick	Breastfeeding is generally safe when mothers have mild illnesses. Infections are rarely transmitted through breast milk, and continued breastfeeding can offer antibodies to the baby. However, serious illnesses may require temporary cessation or precautions.
Myth #5: Breastfeeding is instinctual and easy	Breastfeeding can be challenging as both mother and baby need time to adjust. Issues like low milk supply, latch problems, or discomfort are common and may require support and learning. Education and assistance can greatly improve the breastfeeding experience.
Myth #6: Baby bump disappears immediately after childbirth	The uterus takes time to shrink after childbirth, and abdominal muscles need recovery. The baby bump doesn't disappear instantly but gradually reduces over weeks to months with proper postpartum care and physical activity. Expecting immediate flattening can lead to unrealistic expectations.
Myth #7: Postpartum depression is universal	Postpartum depression is not experienced by all mothers; it affects a minority. It's important to distinguish between postpartum blues (temporary mood swings) and depression (more prolonged and severe). Awareness and support can help manage postpartum emotional challenges effectively.
Myth #8: Breastfeeding preventsm pregnancy	While exclusive breastfeeding can delay fertility (lactational amenorrhoea), it's not a foolproof contraceptive method. Mothers can ovulate and conceive while breastfeeding, so using contraception is still advised to prevent unintended pregnancies.

Beyond this we can also talk about these common questions that new mothers often ask me.

Q: Is it important to have someone nearby for the first 24 hours after delivery?

A: The first 24 hours after delivery are critical for both the mother and the baby. Having a trusted person nearby provides physical and emotional support, helps monitor the mother's recovery and the baby's well-being, assists with baby care, ensures the mother gets rest, and recognizes any signs of complications that may need urgent medical attention.

Q: What is normal postpartum bleeding and lochia?

A: Postpartum bleeding, known as lochia, is normal and can last for up to six weeks. The flow is typically heavy for the first few days, then gradually decreases. It should change from red to pink or brown and finally to yellowish-white. If the bleeding becomes very heavy (soaking a pad in an hour), contains large clots, or has a foul odor, seek medical care urgently.

Q: What are the danger signs for the mother during the postpartum period?

A: Key danger signs include:

- **Severe Bleeding (Hemorrhage):** Soaking through more than one sanitary pad per hour, large blood clots, or continuous bright red bleeding beyond the first few days.
- **High Fever (Infection):** A fever of 100.4°F (38°C) or higher, chills, or flu-like symptoms.
- **Foul-Smelling Discharge:** A strong, unpleasant odor from vaginal discharge or lochia.
- **Severe Headache or Visual Disturbances:** Intense,

persistent headaches, blurred vision, or seeing spots.

- **Severe Abdominal Pain:** Intense, continuous pain in the abdomen, especially with other symptoms like nausea or vomiting.
- **Leg Pain and Swelling (Deep Vein Thrombosis):** Pain, swelling, redness, or warmth in one leg, especially in the calf.

Q: How can new mothers maintain personal hygiene to prevent infections?

A: New mothers should use sanitary pads and change them regularly, wash their hands frequently, and care for any episiotomy or C-section wounds as instructed. Avoid inserting anything into the vagina during the postpartum period.

Q: When can new mothers resume sexual relations and why is birth spacing important?

A: Sexual intercourse should be avoided until any perineal wounds have fully healed. Using condoms is important to prevent STIs and HIV transmission. Discuss family planning methods with your healthcare provider to ensure proper birth spacing, which benefits both maternal and infant health.

Q: What are the key considerations for infant feeding and breast care?

A: Breastfeeding is the optimal way to feed your baby, providing essential nutrients and antibodies. Ensure proper latch and positioning to avoid nipple pain and engorgement. Only take medications prescribed by your healthcare provider, as some can affect breastfeeding.

Q: What is the importance and recommended timing of postnatal visits?

A: Postnatal visits are essential to monitor the health of both the mother and the baby. The first visit should occur within the first week after birth, preferably within 2-3 days, followed by additional visits at 1-2 weeks, 6 weeks, and then as advised by your healthcare provider. These visits help track the baby's development, ensure proper feeding, and monitor the mother's recovery.

Q: Why is it important for new mothers to eat more and healthier foods?

A: Proper nutrition is crucial for a new mother's recovery and for breastfeeding. It's important to eat a balanced diet rich in fruits, vegetables, whole grains, and lean proteins. Drinking plenty of clean, safe water is essential to stay hydrated, especially when breastfeeding.

Chapter 4

UNDERSTANDING YOUR BABY

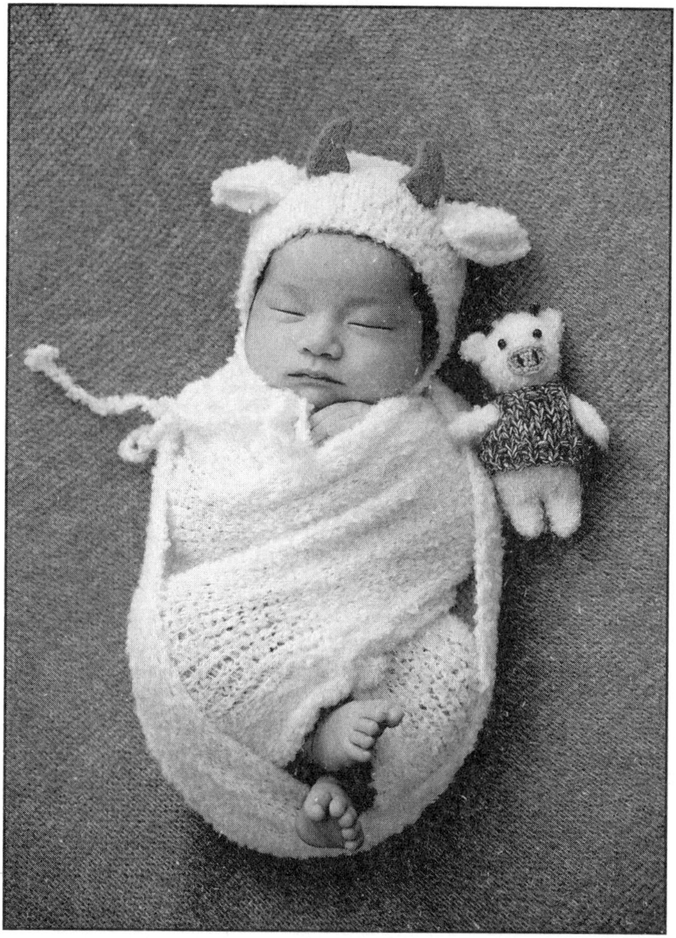

Now that we have talked about your struggles. Let's see what a child actually goes through after coming into this world.

The outside world is a totally new experience for this tiny life. Just moments after leaving the warmth and security of the womb, a baby must cry. In the womb, a baby receives oxygen through the placenta and umbilical cord, not using their lungs to breathe. The first cry helps expand the baby's lungs and clears any amniotic fluid from their airways, initiating the breathing process. This cry signals that the baby's respiratory system is functioning and they are taking in oxygen on their own.

As they take their first breaths, their lungs fill with air, and they experience a rush of sensations—bright lights, unfamiliar sounds, and the sensation of being gently handled by caring hands. This transition from the womb to the outside world is both amazing and overwhelming.

From the very beginning, a newborn's senses are active and alert. While their vision is initially blurry, they can detect light and movement. They are particularly drawn to faces and high-contrast patterns, like black and white shapes. Over time, their vision sharpens, allowing them to focus better on objects and people around them.

Newborns have a keen sense of hearing from the start. They recognize familiar voices they've heard while in the womb, such as their parents' voices. Sounds are not only heard but felt; they can sense vibrations through their bodies, adding another layer to their sensory experience.

Touch is incredibly important for a newborn. They are sensitive to temperature changes and the feeling of being held close. Skin-to-skin contact with their parents not only comforts them but also helps regulate their body temperature and heart rate. Gentle touches and caresses are soothing and reassuring to them in this new world.

At birth, a baby's reflexes are fully functional. They instinctively grasp onto fingers placed in their hands (the palmar grasp reflex) and will turn their head towards anything that strokes their cheek (the rooting reflex), which helps them find the breast for feeding.

Emotionally, newborns seek comfort and security. They may cry to communicate their needs–whether they're hungry, uncomfortable, or just want to be held close to feel safe. Being close to their caregivers provides them with the reassurance they need as they adjust to life outside the womb.

Baby's Developmental Stages (0-1 Years)

The first year of a baby's life is filled with remarkable growth and developmental milestones. Understanding these stages helps parents and caregivers provide the necessary support for their baby's physical, emotional, and cognitive development. However, remember these stages are fluid and not rigid, these are not exact timelines, but based upon largely observed data.

1. Newborn Stage (0-3 Months)

First month

- bringing hands and fists toward mouth (though not always with great accuracy)
- developing reflexes – flinching at loud sounds, shutting eyes at bright lights
- focusing on objects brought within 12 feet of their face
- turning toward familiar sounds and voices – like yours!

Second month

- gurgling/cooing
- trying to follow movement with their eyes (called tracking), although it may not seem very coordinated
- holding their head up and pushing upward with their arms while lying on their tummy

Third Month

- smiling at the sound of your voice (pro tip: record this and review in 15 years to prove that there was once a time your child liked you)
- holding their head and chest up and kicking their legs when lying on their stomach
- grasping toys
- putting their hand in their mouth with more precision
- making more vowel sounds (ooh and ah)
- recognizing familiar faces and objects from a distance
- trying to imitate your facial expressions

2. **Infant Stage (4-6 Months)**

Fourth Month

- holding a rattle and shaking it at the same time
- perhaps starting to roll from tummy to back
- tracking movement more fluidly
- pushing down on legs when held in standing position

Fifth Month

- rolling from tummy to back and then back to tummy
- grabbing their feet, and maybe even inserting them into their mouth
- moving objects from one hand to another

- showing interest in the food you're eating, a sign they're getting ready for solid foods

Sixth Month

- sitting up briefly without any support
- saying consonant (mmmm) and vowel (eeee, ooooo) sounds
- playing and expressing displeasure when playtime stops (keep those raspberries coming!)
- trying to get things that are out of reach
- recognizing their name
- expressing emotion (by crying or whining when sad or angry and laughing or squealing when happy)

3. Older Infant Stage (7-9 Months)

Seventh Month

- sitting up without support for longer periods
- responding to the word "no"
- recognizing emotions (happy, stern, etc.) by your tone
- using their hand like a rake to reach for something (called the "raking grasp")
- responding to expressions — smiling at a smiling face, looking uncertain at a fearful one
- putting objects in their mouth to explore them (parenting tip #204: keep all garbage cans — and, for the love of all things sacred, diaper pails! — in a locked position; you'll thank us later)
- tracking objects more smoothly
- stringing more consonants together while babbling

Eighth Month

- rocking back and forth on their hands and knees or scoot along the floor (precursors to crawling)

- pulling up to a standing position
- drooling – a lot (some babies will be cutting their first teeth around this age)
- continuing to babble (was that a random ma-ma or da-da you just heard?!)
- developing stranger or separation anxiety – this is a kind of distress babies feel when they're separated from their parents or primary caregivers

Don't worry – separation anxiety passes. We promise you'll eventually be able to go to the bathroom alone again.

Ninth Month

- crawling
- more confidently pulling up to a standing position
- playing peekaboo or looking for an object you've hidden
- using the pincer grip (which involves holding a small object like a piece of cereal or pasta between their forefinger and thumb)
- pointing at things they want

4. Late Infant Stage (10-11 Months)

Tenth Month

- moving from pulling to stand or crawling to "cruising," or walking while holding on to furniture or objects around a room
- banging objects together just to hear the sound they make – a kind of auditory assault rivaled only by your neighbor's garage band
- poking at things
- putting objects into a container and then taking them out again

- feeding themselves finger foods
- shaking their head "no" and waving "bye-bye"

Eleventh Month

- continuing to explore language, giving you more mamas, dadas, and maybe even the occasional uh-oh! using the right inflection
- understanding simple declarative statements, such as "don't touch"
- copying your behaviors, like pushing buttons on a play phone and babbling to mimic conversation

5. **One-Year-Old (12 Months)**

Physical Development:

- Most babies can stand alone and may begin walking unassisted.
- Improved hand-eye coordination; starts to stack blocks and use objects like spoons.

Cognitive Development:

- Demonstrates understanding of simple concepts like in and out, or open and close.
- Begins to show memory of people, places, and objects from previous experiences.

Emotional And Social Development:

- Shows signs of independence, such as wanting to feed themselves.
- Enjoys playing alongside other children (parallel play) but may not yet engage in cooperative play.

Twelfth Month

- cruising, standing briefly unsupported, and maybe even

taking a step or two
- exploring objects by banging, throwing, and dropping them
- saying one or two simple words, such as hi, no, and bye
- using objects correctly, if not clumsily (for example, using a spoon to eat and a comb to brush hair)
- looking to the right object when you say, "Where's the dog?" or "Where's grandma?"

Supporting Baby's Development

Parents and caregivers play a crucial role in supporting their baby's development through:

- Responding to the baby's needs promptly and lovingly.
- Providing a safe space for exploration and play.
- Ensuring the baby receives appropriate nutrition for their age.
- Engaging in activities that stimulate their senses and encourage movement and interaction.
- Regular pediatric check-ups to monitor growth and development and address any concerns.

Chapter 5

A GUIDE TO HAPPY BABIES AND HEALTHY MOTHERS

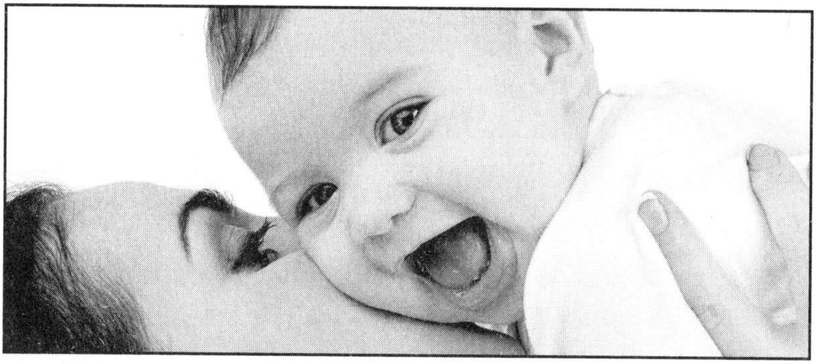

Now that you know the developmental stages of your child and the expected stages of your transition to motherhood, let's explore the intersection of both of your journeys together.

In this chapter I am adding some of the topics that new mothers have most questions about. These topics are consolidated into broader themes.

1. Breastfeeding

Breastfeeding is a natural process, it is nature's preparation to provide for the baby who is too young to taste and digest the food that we take as our meals.

Breast milk offers immense benefits for both baby and a mother. Breast milk is often referred to as nature's perfect food for infants. It is rich in vital nutrients, antibodies, and enzymes specifically designed to meet the needs of a growing baby. The first milk, known as colostrum, is especially beneficial, packed with immune-boosting properties that protect newborns from infections and illnesses. As the baby grows, the composition of breast milk adapts to meet their changing nutritional requirements, making it an invaluable source of nourishment throughout infancy.

For mothers, breastfeeding offers numerous health benefits. It aids in postpartum recovery by helping the uterus return to its pre-pregnancy size and reducing postpartum bleeding. Long-term, breastfeeding is associated with a lower risk of breast and ovarian cancers, as well as cardiovascular diseases. Additionally, the act of breastfeeding releases oxytocin, a hormone that promotes relaxation and emotional well-being.

Breastfeeding also promotes emotional bonding and security. The close physical contact during breastfeeding fosters a sense of warmth and comfort, helping to build a strong and loving connection between mother and baby.

Mothers have a lot of questions related to Breastfeeding and for the sake of a better understanding, I am presenting it in Q&A format.

Q1: How soon after birth should I start breastfeeding my baby?

A1: It's best to start breastfeeding within the first hour after birth if possible. This helps initiate bonding and stimulates milk production. The first milk, called colostrum, is rich in nutrients and antibodies, providing essential protection for your newborn.

Q2: How often should I breastfeed my newborn?

A2: Newborns typically need to feed every 1 to 4 hours, which means about 8-12 times in 24 hours. Frequent feeding helps establish your milk supply and ensures your baby gets enough nutrients for growth.

Feeding Frequency

- **Initial Phase (Newborns):**
  - ❖ **Frequency:** Every 1-4 hours
  - ❖ **Method:** Demand feeding (feeding as per the baby's demand)
- **First week of life:**
  - ❖ **Frequency:** 6-9 feeds per day
- **9-12 Months of age:**
  - ❖ **Frequency:** 3-5 meals per day

Q3: How can I tell if my baby is getting enough milk?

A3: Signs that your baby is getting enough milk include:

- Regular weight gain (your pediatrician will monitor this).

- Six or more wet diapers a day by the time they are a week old.
- Regular bowel movements.
- Baby seems satisfied and content after feeding.
- You can hear or see your baby swallowing during feeds.

Q4: What should I do if breastfeeding is painful?

A4: Breastfeeding shouldn't be painful. If you're experiencing pain, it might be due to incorrect latch or positioning. Make sure your baby's mouth covers a large part of the areola, not just the nipple. Consult a lactation consultant or your pediatrician for guidance. They can help adjust your technique and address any issues such as nipple soreness or engorgement.

Q5: Can I breastfeed if I have to return to work?

A5: Absolutely! You can continue breastfeeding by expressing milk and storing it for your baby. Invest in a good quality breast pump and establish a pumping schedule that mimics your baby's feeding pattern. Properly stored breast milk can be kept in the refrigerator for up to 4 days or in the freezer for about 6 months.

Q6: What foods should I avoid while breastfeeding?

A6: Most foods are safe while breastfeeding, but some may cause issues like gas or fussiness in your baby. Common culprits can include caffeine, spicy foods, and certain vegetables like broccoli or cabbage. If you notice a pattern, you might try eliminating that food to see if it helps. However, maintaining a balanced and nutritious diet is key.

Q7: How long should I breastfeed my baby?

A7: Exclusive breastfeeding is recommended for the first six months. After that, you can continue breastfeeding while introducing solid foods. The World Health Organization recommends breastfeeding along with complementary foods up to 2 years of age or beyond, depending on mutual desire.

Q8: How do I position my baby for breastfeeding?

A8: Proper positioning and attachment are crucial for effective breastfeeding. During breastfeeding, the infant's head, neck, and body should be held in a straight line, ensuring that the whole body is supported, not just the head and neck. The baby's face should be directly in front of the mother's breast, and the baby's body should be close to the mother's body to facilitate a comfortable and secure latch.

For proper attachment, the baby's chin should touch the breast, and the mouth should be wide open. The baby's lower lip should be turned out, and most of the areola and nipple should be in the baby's mouth. It's important that more of the areola is visible above the baby's mouth than below, ensuring a deep latch that helps the baby feed efficiently and reduces discomfort for the mother.

Q9: What should I do if I can't produce enough milk?

A9: If you're concerned about your milk supply, ensure frequent and effective breastfeeding or pumping sessions to stimulate production. Stay hydrated, eat a balanced diet, and get enough rest. If the issue persists, consult your pediatrician or a lactation consultant. They can provide strategies to boost milk production or explore supplementing options if necessary.

Breastfeeding can be a rewarding experience for both you and your baby. Remember, every mother and baby are unique, so what works for one may not work for another. Don't hesitate to seek support from healthcare professionals and lactation consultants along the way.

To Summarize:

Breastfeeding offers the best nutrition for your baby and helps build immunity. Aim to breastfeed exclusively for the first six months if possible. Breast milk is the best milk till 6 months of age. However, if due to any reasons the mother is not able to produce breast milk, the second choice should be formula feed. A child should never be given cow milk, goat milk or any other type of animal milk, because the human body especially at a newborn stage is not at all efficient in digesting it or extracting any nutrition out of it. The protein composition in human milk is predominantly whey, with a casein-to-whey ratio of approximately 40:60 in early lactation, shifting to about 50:50 later on. Whey proteins are easily digestible and help support the infant's digestive system and rapid growth. In contrast, cow's milk has a higher casein content, with a casein-to-whey ratio of about 80:20. The higher casein level makes cow's milk more difficult for infants to digest and can lead to gastrointestinal discomfort. Human milk is high in lactose, providing a key energy source and aiding calcium absorption, and contains vital vitamins and minerals in highly bioavailable forms. Unlike cow's milk, which has higher protein levels that can be hard for infants to digest, and lacks the immunological components necessary for protecting infants from infections, human milk offers antibodies, white blood cells, and other immunological factors that bolster an infant's developing immune system. While cow's milk and other animal milks, such as goat's and sheep's milk, are used to make infant formulas, they must be significantly modified to resemble the nutrient profile of human milk.

2. Weaning

Starting Weaning At 6 Months

Weaning aims to gradually introduce your baby to a broader range of foods and textures so that by the age of 1 year, they can participate in family meals. Babies develop at different paces—some may adapt quickly to new foods, while others might need more time or multiple exposures to accept new tastes.

When To Introduce Solid Foods

According to the latest research, babies only need breastmilk or infant formula for the first six months. This is because their digestive systems and kidneys are still maturing. Introducing solids too early can increase the risk of asthma, eczema, digestive issues, allergies, and obesity later in life.

Although every baby is different, there are three clear signs that indicate readiness for solid foods alongside breast milk or infant formula:

1. The baby can sit up and hold their head steady.
2. The baby can coordinate their eyes, hands, and mouth to look at food, pick it up, and put it in their mouth independently.
3. The baby can swallow food (a baby who isn't ready will push food back out of their mouth).

There isn't a perfect time of day to introduce the first solid foods; instead, choose a calm moment when your baby isn't too hungry. Offer a small amount of food either before or after a milk feed, or even during the feed if that works best. Keep in mind that not all foods need to be spoon-fed—your baby can start feeding themselves with their hands as soon as they show interest.

It's normal if your baby initially rejects solid foods. Don't be discouraged—try again at the next mealtime. The main goal at this stage is to help your baby get used to different tastes and textures. If using a spoon, wait until your baby opens their mouth before offering food. Start with just a few teaspoons of food once a day. Your baby may also enjoy holding a spoon and mimicking others.

Continue providing the usual amount of breastmilk or infant formula, as it will still be the primary source of nourishment during the early stages of weaning.

Complementary Feeding (Weaning)

Age	Liquid	Semi Liquid	Semi Solid	Solid
6 Months	Thin purees - apple, pear. Juices- apple, carrot. Soups- carrot, bottle gourd, tomato, spinach, pumpkin, beet. Dal, not very dilute Rice Kanji			
	2 Times a day (11 am, 4 pm)			

Age	Liquid	Semi Liquid	Semi Solid	Solid
	90-100 ml			
	Breast or formula feeds as needed			
7 Months		Porridges - suji, oats, ragi, daliya, sabudana, wheat with milk/water. Halwa with carrot, beet. Khichdi with more dal. Mixed vegetable soup carrot, potato, pumpkin, Thick Fruit purees: banana, mango papaya, chiku. Curd/butter milk		
		3 Times a day (11 am, 4 pm, 8 am)		
		100-200 ml		
		Milk - 4-5 Times a day		

Age	Liquid	Semi Liquid	Semi Solid	Solid
8-10 Months			Boiled/cooked mashed vegetables. Boiled potato, sweet potato, Thick khichdi. Mashed banana, chiku. Mashed roti in dal, Egg yolk. Finger foods by 9 months. Well cooked sticks of vegetables, cheese, potato, paneer.	
			4 Times a day	
			Up to 250 ml	
			Breast or formula milk 3-4 Times a day	
11-12 Months				Complete family food well cooked, chopped.
				5-6 Times a day
				Milk 2-3 Times a day

https://www.publichealth.hscni.net/sites/default/files/2019-03/Weaning_made_easy_nov%202018_0.pdf

Precautions:**

- **No Salt/Sugar/Chilli/Spices:** Avoid adding these to the baby's food as their kidneys are not yet mature enough to process high levels of salt, and sugar can contribute to unhealthy weight gain and dental issues.
- **Follow the 3-Day Rule:** Introduce one new food at a time and wait for three days before introducing another to monitor for any allergic reactions.
- **Increasing Calorie Density:** Add ghee, butter, or oil to foods to increase their calorie content, especially if the baby is not gaining weight as expected.
- **Dry Fruits Powder:** Can be used to improve calorie density once the baby is accustomed to semi-solid and solid foods.
- **Introducing Cow Milk:** Cow's milk can be introduced after 1 year of age, but it should not replace breast milk or formula until then.

Practical Tips:

- Maintain a consistent feeding schedule to help establish routine.
- Ensure all utensils and food preparation areas are clean to prevent infections.
- Be patient and offer new foods multiple times, as babies may need to try a new food several times before accepting it.

3. Baby Cues (0-1 Years)

Understanding baby cues is a big puzzle that new parents struggle the most with. Babies communicate through a range of nonverbal cues that signal their needs and emotional states. Recognizing these cues can help parents provide appropriate care and comfort.

Hunger Cues

Early Signs:

- When a baby turns their head toward anything that strokes their cheek or mouth, it's a sign they are looking for food.
- Babies often suck on their hands or fingers when they are hungry. This is a natural reflex that helps them calm down and signal hunger.
- Smacking lips or making sucking noises are also indicators of hunger.

Late Signs:

- Crying is a late hunger cue. By the time a baby starts crying, they may already be quite hungry. Early recognition of hunger cues can prevent the baby from becoming overly distressed (AAP Pediatrics in Review) (AAP Publications).

Tiredness Cues

Common Signs:

- Babies often rub their eyes when they are tired.
- Just like adults, babies yawn when they are sleepy.
- Increased fussiness or irritability can indicate that a baby needs to sleep. They might also pull at their ears or have trouble focusing.

Overt Signs:

- Slowing down in activity or becoming less engaged with surroundings can be a sign of tiredness.
- Turning away from engaging activities or people can signal that a baby needs rest (**AAP Pediatrics in Review) (AAP Publications**).

Overstimulation Cues

Indicators:

- When overstimulated, babies may turn their heads away from lights, sounds, or people.
- Arching their back and stiffening their body can be a response to too much stimulation.
- Persistent crying, even after being fed and changed, can indicate that the baby is overwhelmed by their environment.

Calming Strategies:

- Reducing noise and visual stimulation can help soothe an overstimulated baby.
- Swaddling can provide a sense of security and comfort, helping to calm the baby down **(AAP Publications) (AAP Publications)**.

Understanding And Responding To Baby Cues

Spend time observing your baby to learn their specific cues and patterns. Each baby is unique and may express their needs differently. Responding consistently to your baby's cues helps them feel secure and understood. Establishing a daily routine can help anticipate and meet your baby's needs before they become distressed.

By paying close attention to these cues, parents can better meet their baby's needs, ensuring that they feel safe, secure, and loved. Early intervention and attentive caregiving are key to fostering a nurturing environment for infants **(AAP Pediatrics in Review) (AAP Publications) (AAP Publications)**.

4. Speech Development

Talking to your baby from day one supports speech

development. Respond to their coos and babbles, read to them, and describe your actions. By 6-12 months, babies may start saying simple words like "mama" and "dada."

Speech development in infants during the first year is a fascinating and vital process. Babies progress through several key milestones as they begin to understand and produce language. By third year you can expect them to speak fluently with a good vocabulary.

Birth to 3 Months

- Newborns start to coo and make gurgling sounds. These are early forms of vocal play that help them explore their vocal range.
- Babies use different cries to signal hunger, discomfort, or tiredness. Parents often start to distinguish between these cries over time.
- Infants react to loud noises by startling or becoming quiet. They also begin to recognize familiar voices, particularly those of their parents.

4 To 6 Months

- Around this age, babies begin to laugh and giggle, which are signs of joy and social engagement.
- They start to mimic facial expressions and sounds, demonstrating early social interaction skills.
- Babies experiment with sounds, combining consonants and vowels in repetitive sequences like "ba-ma" or "da-da" (ASHA) (Stanford Children's).

7 To 9 Months

- Babies begin to respond to their names and can turn towards the person calling them.

- They start to babble, using varied intonation that mimics the patterns of speech.
- Infants begin to understand basic words like "no" and "bye-bye," and might even try to mimic them (Mayo Clinic).

10 To 12 Months

- Typically, by their first birthday, babies may say one or two words such as "mama" or "dada" with meaning.
- They can follow simple instructions, especially when accompanied by gestures, such as "come here."
- Babies try to imitate the sounds and words they hear from adults, an essential step in language development (NIDCD) (ASHA).

13 Months:

- 2-3 recognizable words

14-15 Months:

- 2-6 recognizable words
- Can name a familiar object (e.g., pencil)

15-16 Months:

- Uses childhood jargon
- Can name pictures

18 Months:

- Many intelligible words
- Speaks at least 6 words
- Uses 6-20 recognizable words (about 18 words)
- Points to eye, nose, ear
- Attempts to sing a song

2 Years:

- Says simple 2-word sentences

- Repeats things said
- Uses me, I, you
- Speaks 50 or more words
- Understands 120-175 words
- Points to at least one part of the body

2.5 Years (30 Months):

- Joins in nursery rhymes and sings
- Puts 2-3 words into simple sentences
- Phrases of 2-3 words
- Asks names of objects/people
- Uses pronouns, prepositions
- Understands 400 words

3 Years (36 Months):

- Good vocabulary of 250 or more words
- Understands 800 words, uses plurals
- Asks questions
- 3-6 word sentences

Supporting Speech Development

You can narrate your activities and describe what you see throughout the day. This constant exposure to language helps babies learn. Reading books, even simple picture books, introduces babies to new words and concepts. Singing songs with repetitive phrases and melodies can captivate babies and reinforce language patterns. When your baby makes sounds, respond and imitate them. This back-and-forth interaction encourages them to continue experimenting with their voice.

When To Seek Help

If you notice that your baby isn't meeting these milestones, it may be beneficial to consult a healthcare provider. Factors such as hearing issues or developmental delays can impact speech development, and early intervention can be crucial. Specialists like audiologists and speech-language pathologists can offer assessments and guidance (Mayo Clinic)(Stanford Children's).

5. Crawling And Walking

Crawling Stage

Crawling typically begins around 6-10 months. Create a safe space for your baby to explore. Encourage crawling by placing toys just out of reach and providing lots of tummy time.

The crawling stage is a critical milestone in a baby's motor development, typically occurring between 6 to 10 months of age. This stage marks the transition from stationary sitting or lying down to actively moving around on all fours, preparing infants for further exploration and interaction with their environment.

Crawling plays a crucial role in strengthening muscles and refining coordination. Research suggests that crawling helps develop cross-pattern movements, which are important for brain development and future motor skills like walking and running (Kuo, 2018). As babies crawl, they learn to navigate their surroundings, enhancing spatial perception and depth perception (Adolph & Berger, 2015). The act of crawling involves problem-solving skills as babies strategize to reach objects, promoting cognitive development and spatial reasoning (Anderson et al., 2020).

Creating A Safe Environment

1. It's essential to create a safe space for crawling babies by removing hazards, ensuring electrical outlets are covered, and securing furniture that could be pulled down.

2. Placing toys just out of reach encourages babies to crawl towards them, fostering motivation and physical activity. Tummy time helps strengthen muscles needed for crawling (Majnemer & Barr, 2006).

Parental Guidance And Support

While the timing of crawling varies, parents should monitor their baby's progress and consult healthcare providers if there are concerns about motor development delays.

The crawling stage is an exciting time in a baby's life, marking significant progress in motor, cognitive, and spatial development. By creating a safe and stimulating environment and encouraging exploration, parents can support their baby's journey towards greater independence and physical competence.

During the crawling stage, babies rely on various supports to facilitate their exploration and development of motor skills. However, it's important to take care of certain aspects during this stage.

Do's:

1. Create a safe and spacious area free from hazards such as sharp objects, electrical cords, and small items that could be choking hazards. Use soft mats or carpets to cushion falls.
2. Encourage tummy time from an early age to help strengthen neck, shoulder, and arm muscles, which are crucial for crawling. Start with short sessions and gradually increase time as your baby grows more comfortable.
3. Place toys and objects just out of reach to motivate your baby to crawl towards them. These stimuli encourage movement and exploration, promoting both physical and cognitive

development.

4. Supervise your baby during crawling practice to ensure their safety and provide encouragement. Stay nearby to offer support and assistance if needed, but allow them to explore independently as much as possible.
5. Praise your baby's efforts and milestones in crawling. Positive reinforcement helps build confidence and motivation to continue exploring their environment.

Don'ts:

1. While some babies may use knee pads for protection, avoid overly restricting their movement with tight clothing or accessories that could hinder natural crawling motions.
2. Every baby develops at their own pace. Avoid forcing your baby into crawling positions or pushing them to move faster than they are ready for. Let them progress naturally through the stages of motor development.
3. While devices like playpens or baby gates can provide a safe space, avoid confining your baby for extended periods. Babies need opportunities to move freely and develop their motor skills.
4. Allow your baby to explore different surfaces and textures during crawling. Restricting exploration could hinder sensory development and curiosity.
5. Ensure that the crawling area is free of hazards such as stairs, sharp edges, or unstable furniture. Supervision is crucial to prevent accidents and injuries.

By providing a supportive environment and following these do's and don'ts, parents can encourage and nurture their baby's natural curiosity and development during the crawling stage.

Walking Stage

Most babies start walking between 9-15 months. Offer support by holding their hands. Ensure the environment is safe for exploration.

The walking stage in infants marks a significant developmental milestone, typically occurring between 9 to 15 months of age. This period is characterized by babies transitioning from crawling or cruising (walking while holding onto furniture) to walking independently.

Walking requires coordination of multiple muscle groups, including those in the legs, hips, and core. As babies practice walking, they strengthen these muscles, improving overall motor skills (Adolph & Robinson, 2015). Learning to balance while walking helps babies develop better posture and spatial awareness. This skill is crucial for their physical development and future motor activities (Thelen, 1995). Walking fosters cognitive development by enhancing spatial reasoning and problem-solving abilities. It also facilitates social interactions as babies explore their environment more independently (Clearfield, 2011).

Supportive Measures

1. Providing physical support by holding your baby's hands or under their arms helps them feel secure and maintain balance as they practice walking. This support encourages confidence and reduces the risk of falls (Ivanenko et al., 2013).
2. Ensuring a safe environment is critical during the walking stage. Remove obstacles, secure furniture that could be pulled down, and use safety gates to prevent access to stairs

or other hazardous areas (Shields, 2013).

Parental Guidance

1. Every baby develops at their own pace. Encourage your baby's efforts with positive reinforcement and celebrate their progress. Be patient and supportive as they gain confidence in their walking abilities (Piek et al., 2010).
2. While the typical range for walking onset is 9-15 months, consult with healthcare providers if you have concerns about delays or motor development issues. Early intervention can sometimes be beneficial if there are developmental concerns (Campbell & Eaton, 2019).

The walking stage is an exciting time in a baby's life, representing a major achievement in motor and cognitive development. By providing supportive measures, a safe environment, and parental guidance, parents can help their babies navigate this stage with confidence and foster healthy physical and cognitive growth.

Supports used during walking for babies typically involve aids that provide stability and balance as they develop their walking skills. However, don't forget to take care of these aspects.

Dos:

1. Holding your baby's hands or providing support under their arms can help them maintain balance and gain confidence in their walking abilities.
2. When babies start walking outside or on hard surfaces, soft-soled shoes can protect their feet while allowing them to feel the ground and maintain balance.

3. Ensure the walking area is free of hazards and obstacles that could cause tripping or falling. Provide a clear, open space for your baby to practice walking.
4. Encourage your baby with positive reinforcement and praise. Celebrate their efforts and achievements in walking to boost their confidence.

Don'ts:

1. Walkers with wheels can be dangerous as they allow babies to move too quickly and potentially reach hazardous areas or fall down stairs. It's safer to use stationary or push walkers. These may also eat away on the child's confidence to do the task on their own.
2. Every baby develops at their own pace. Avoid pushing or forcing your baby to walk before they are physically ready. Let them progress naturally through crawling and cruising stages.
3. While walking toys can be entertaining, they don't provide the support needed for learning to walk and can interfere with the development of proper walking skills.
4. Ensure that your baby walks on safe, flat surfaces. Avoid surfaces that are slippery or uneven, as they can increase the risk of falls and injuries.
5. While support is beneficial, excessive assistance may hinder your baby's ability to develop balance and coordination independently. Gradually reduce support as your baby gains confidence and stability.

References:

- Adolph, K. E., & Robinson, S. R. (2015). Motor Development.

In M. H. Bornstein & T. Leventhal (Eds.), Handbook of Child Psychology and Developmental Science (7th ed., Vol. 2, pp. 1-45). John Wiley & Sons.

- Clearfield, M. W. (2011). Learning to Walk Changes Infants' Social Interactions. Infant Behavior and Development, 34(1), 15-25.
- Ivanenko, Y. P., Dominici, N., Cappellini, G., Dan, B., Cheron, G., & Lacquaniti, F. (2013). Development of pendulum mechanism and kinematic coordination from the first unsupported steps in toddlers. Journal of Experimental Biology, 216(21), 3915-3923.
- Piek, J. P., Dawson, L., Smith, L. M., & Gasson, N. (2010). The role of early fine and gross motor development on later motor and cognitive ability. Human Movement Science, 29(4), 604-612.
- Wu, Y. H., Wang, M. H., & Su, F. C. (2020). Effects of a push toy on the early walking patterns of toddlers. Gait & Posture, 81, 75-80.

6. Bathing And Massages

According to guidelines from the American Academy of Pediatrics and research published in Pediatrics, infants should be bathed daily for hygiene and to maintain skin health. However, for the first 10 days after birth, sponge bathing is recommended to protect the umbilical cord stump until it falls off naturally (Johnston et al., 2016). During sponge bathing, gently cleanse your baby's face, hands, and diaper area using a soft washcloth or sponge. Avoid immersing the baby in water until the umbilical cord stump has healed and fallen off to prevent infection (American Academy of Pediatrics,

2020). Light massages can be beneficial for soothing infants and promoting relaxation. Use gentle, circular motions with a small amount of baby-safe oil or lotion, focusing on areas like the back, arms, and legs. When selecting oils or lotions for massages, opt for products specifically formulated for babies to avoid irritation or allergic reactions. Commonly recommended oils include almond oil, coconut oil, or hypoallergenic baby oils that are free of fragrances and additives (Feldman et al., 2002). Research shows benefits for light massages, rigorous motions and scrubbing can harm the skin of the baby as it is very sensitive during the initial years.

Practical Tips

- Ensure the room is comfortably warm before undressing your baby for bathing or massages. Use mild, fragrance-free baby soap and shampoo designed for delicate skin.
- Handle your baby with care during bathing and massages to prevent accidents or discomfort. Support their head and neck when lifting or moving them.
- Observe your baby's reactions during massages and adjust techniques if they seem uncomfortable. Massages should be enjoyable and relaxing experiences for both the baby and parent.

Note:

In many cultures including Indian, the arrival of a new baby is accompanied by the tradition of baby massages performed by a "dai ma" or caregiver. While these practices are deeply rooted in cultural beliefs, their purported benefits, such as strengthening bones, lack conclusive scientific evidence.

Modern medical advice encourages parents to continue

these traditions cautiously. Light massages with baby-safe virgin oils, free from adulterants, can provide a soothing experience for infants. This gentle touch not only fosters bonding between the caregiver and the baby but also promotes relaxation.

Despite the lack of scientific backing for claims of bone strengthening, the practice of baby massages remains a cherished tradition in many households.

References:

- American Academy of Pediatrics. (2020). Bathing Your Newborn. Retrieved from https://www.healthychildren.org/English/ages-stages/baby/bathing-skin-care/Pages/Bathing-Your-Newborn.aspx
- Feldman, R., Rosenthal, Z., & Eidelman, A. I. (2002). Maternal-preterm skin-to-skin contact enhances child physiologic organization and cognitive control across the first 10 years of life. Biological Psychiatry, 74(11), 863-871.
- Field, T. (2010). Postnatal depression effects on early interactions, parenting, and safety practices: A review. Infant Behavior and Development, 33(1), 1-6.
- Johnston, S., Baez, M. V., & Amoa, A. (2016). The use of infant massage in a case of child neglect. Pediatrics, 138(1), e20154276.

Clothing And Covering

Choose soft, breathable fabrics such as cotton for your baby's clothing. These materials help regulate body temperature and minimize the risk of skin irritation. Avoid synthetic fabrics that may trap heat or cause discomfort (American Academy of Pediatrics, 2020). Dress your baby in layers that can be easily adjusted to maintain comfort in varying temperatures.

This approach allows you to add or remove clothing as needed without overheating or chilling your baby. Adjust clothing choices based on the weather. In cooler temperatures, use lightweight layers under a warm outer layer. In hot weather, dress your baby in lightweight, loose-fitting clothing to promote airflow and prevent overheating.

Diapers

Modern diapers are highly absorbent, which helps keep the baby's skin dry and reduces the risk of diaper rash and infections. A dry diaper can also help babies sleep better and for longer periods. However, there is no harm in using diapers. You should take care that diapers are made from soft, breathable materials. Avoid those with harsh chemicals or fragrances that might irritate the baby's skin. Change diapers frequently to keep the baby's skin dry and prevent diaper rash. Newborns typically need changing every 2-3 hours. Also Ensure that diapers do not restrict your baby's movement or circulation. Check for a snug but not tight fit around the waist and legs to prevent leaks or discomfort.

References:

- American Academy of Pediatrics. (2020). Choosing Safe Baby Products: Cribs. Retrieved from https://www.healthychildren.org/English/safety-prevention/at-home/Pages/Clothing-and-Accessories.aspx
- AAP News. (2019). Diaper dermatitis: Clinical and economic implications. AAP News, 40(1), e20154276.
- Blume-Peytavi, U., Lavender, T., Jenerowicz, D., Ryumina, I., Stalder, J. F., Torrelo, A., & Cork, M. J. (2017). Recommendations from a European roundtable meeting

on best practice healthy infant skin care. Journal of Pediatric Nursing, 36, 28-36.

- Zachariades, F., Oziemski, M., & Bessou-Touya, S. (2014). Management of diaper dermatitis in infants: An exploratory literature review. Pediatrics, 134(3), 436-444.

The first year with your baby is a precious and transformative time. By focusing on both your well-being and your baby's development, you can create a healthy, happy environment. Remember, every baby is different, and trust your instincts as you navigate this journey.

Chapter 6

MYTHS ABOUT BABY CARE DEBUNKED: WHAT ACTUALLY WORKS?

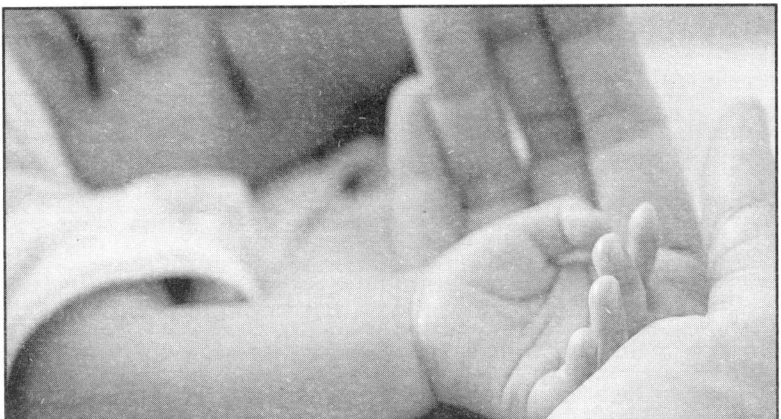

It is crucial for pediatricians to dispel prevalent misconceptions about baby care to prevent hazardous practices. Here is a guide to debunking these myths and understanding proper baby care:

1. Giving Newborns A Bath

- **Myth:** A newborn must be bathed as soon as possible after birth.
- **Fact:** Bathing a newborn immediately can cause hypothermia. Instead, gently sponge them with warm water to clean them without endangering their body temperature.

2. Giving Honey Or Other Sweet Foods To Babies

- **Myth:** Giving a newborn honey or other sweets is good for them.
- **Fact:** This practice poses a risk of botulism. Newborns should be exclusively fed with breast milk or formula for the first six months of life.

3. Baby Massage Oil

- **Myth:** Babies become stronger when they are massaged with oil.
- **Fact:** There is no evidence that massaging babies with oil makes them stronger. Some oils may irritate the skin or cause allergic reactions. Gentle, dry massages can be relaxing without the risks associated with oils. Avoid applying oils to a baby's nose or ears as it can lead to infections and blockages.

4. Sealing The Soft Spot (Fontanelle)

- **Myth:** The fontanelle, or soft spot, will close more quickly if oil is applied there.

- **Fact:** The fontanelle naturally closes on its own between nine and eighteen months. Applying oil is unnecessary and potentially harmful.

5. **Applying Kajal On Eyes**
   - **Myth:** Kajal enlarges and enhances the appearance of the eyes.
   - **Fact:** Kajal, especially homemade, can cause allergic reactions and infections. It is not recommended for young children.

6. **Gram Flour For Fair Skin**
   - **Myth:** A baby's skin becomes fairer after bathing with gram flour.
   - **Fact:** Skin tone is determined by genetics, not external factors. Gram flour can cause allergies and skin issues.

7. **Newborns' Breast Engorgement**
   - **Myth:** Applying pressure to a baby's swollen breasts can reduce swelling and milk production.
   - **Fact:** Breast engorgement in babies is due to maternal hormones and resolves on its own in 4-6 weeks. Pressing can cause infections.

8. **Taking Care Of The Umbilical Cord**
   - **Myth:** Applying oils, ghee, or sindoor to the umbilical cord will help it heal.
   - **Fact:** The umbilical cord should be kept dry and clean until it naturally falls off in 7-10 days.

9. **Summertime Chapped Lips**
   - **Myth:** If a baby's lips are chapped in the summer, they need water.
   - **Fact:** Breast milk provides sufficient hydration for

newborns. Water should not be introduced before six months.

10. Introducing Cow's Milk

- **Myth:** Babies younger than a year old can drink cow's milk.
- **Fact:** Cow's milk can cause protein allergies and is not suitable for babies under a year old.

11. Tying Strings Around Various Body Parts

- **Myth:** Tying threads around a baby's neck, waist, or legs is beneficial.
- **Fact:** This can impair blood flow, cause skin wounds, and induce reactions. It should be avoided.

12. Giving A Child A Cold Bath

- **Myth:** Bathing a child with a cold is not advised.
- **Fact:** Regular baths can be given to a child with a cold without harming their health.

13. Using Air Conditioning

- **Myth:** Babies should not be in air-conditioned rooms.
- **Fact:** Air conditioning can maintain a comfortable temperature. Ensure the baby is adequately dressed and the room is not excessively cold.

14. Applying Moisturizer

- **Myth:** A baby's skin shouldn't be moisturized.
- **Fact:** Moisturizers can be used to keep the skin supple and prevent dryness.

15. Frequency Of Stools

- **Myth:** Infrequent stools indicate a problem.
- **Fact:** It's normal for breastfed infants to have irregular stool patterns. It's normal for a baby to have stools once a

day, once a week, or even every 8-10 days.

16. Teething Timelines

- **Myth:** Teeth should erupt by 7-8 months.
- **Fact:** Teeth typically erupt within the first 1.5 years, but timing varies.

17. Bending Legs

- **Myth:** A baby's curved legs signify a problem.
- **Fact:** Babies often have curled legs due to their position in the womb, and this is normal until about two years old.

18. Nursing The Baby While The Mother Is Ill

- **Myth:** Breastfeeding should stop if the mother is ill.
- **Fact:** Mothers should consult healthcare professionals, but for most illnesses do not require stopping breastfeeding.

19. Colostrum: Busting the Myth of "Cursed Milk" in India

- **Myth:** Colostrum is "cursed milk"
- **Fact:** Colostrum is "liquid gold"

Colostrum, known as "liquid gold," is the first form of milk produced by the mother immediately after childbirth. The World Health Organization (WHO) universally recommends colostrum as the perfect first food for every newborn due to its rich composition of nutrients and antibodies, which are crucial for the baby's immunity, growth, and development.

Despite these benefits, the prevalence of colostrum feeding in India varies significantly, ranging from 21% to 41% across different states.

20. Myth: Breastfeeding Should Be on a Strict Schedule

- **Myth:** Feeding on demand spoils the baby
- **Fact:** Meeting a baby's needs for food and comfort builds trust and security, which are crucial for their development.

Some believe that feeding on demand can spoil the baby or make them too dependent. However, Adhering to a strict feeding schedule can lead to frustration for both the baby and the mother. It can also result in inadequate milk supply and a hungry, fussy baby. Breastfeeding should be based on demand rather than a strict schedule. There can be some routine to it, but creating a rigid time-table will not benefit anyone.

What is on-demand breastfeeding?

On-demand breastfeeding means feeding the baby whenever they show signs of hunger. This could be every 1-3 hours for newborns, as their stomachs are small and they digest breast milk quickly. Babies communicate their hunger through cues such as rooting (turning their head and opening their mouth), sucking on their hands, or becoming more alert and active. Crying is often a late hunger cue. The frequency of breastfeeding can vary widely. Some babies may feed every hour, while others might feed every 2-3 hours. Growth spurts can also increase feeding frequency temporarily.

By debunking these myths and providing information based on professional advice and facts, we can ensure babies receive the best possible care. Always seek advice from medical professionals for any questions regarding baby care.

Chapter 7

DISEASES, DEFICIENCIES (RED SIGNS) AND VACCINES

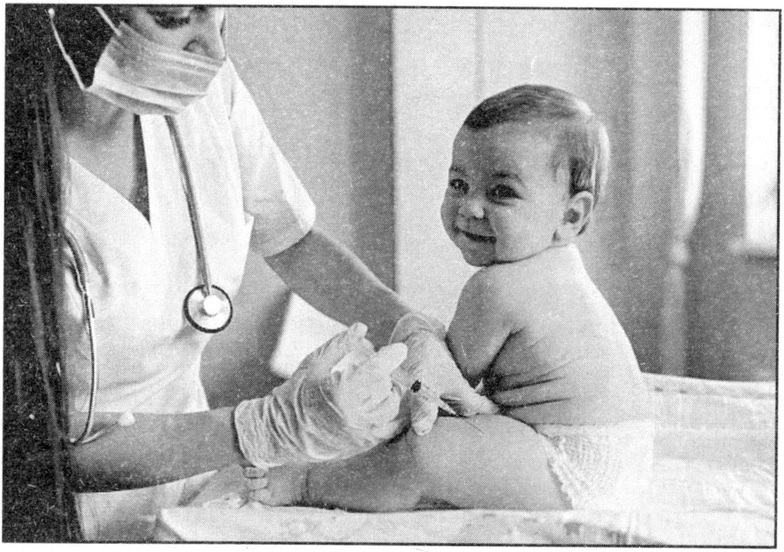

There are countless diseases and deficiencies out there that affect newborns and children. It is not possible and not even necessary to list all of them here. So, instead I am writing about the danger signs and points of consideration to help you to differentiate the normal signs from the Red signals of the onset of diseases and deficiencies.

Diseases

Diseases are conditions that disrupt the normal functioning of the body, resulting in various symptoms and health issues. In newborns, diseases can range from infectious to genetic and metabolic disorders. Infectious diseases, caused by bacteria, viruses, fungi, or parasites, often present with symptoms such as fever, irritability, poor feeding, lethargy, and changes in bowel movements or urination. Genetic disorders, inherited from parents, can lead to a variety of health problems, including metabolic imbalances, developmental delays, and congenital anomalies. Metabolic diseases involve disruptions in the body's chemical processes and can present early in life with symptoms like poor feeding, vomiting, lethargy, and developmental delays. Early detection and treatment are crucial for managing these conditions and minimizing their impact on a newborn's health and development.

Recognizing Normal Behaviors And Development

1. **Feeding:** Newborns typically eat every 2-3 hours. Some variations in appetite are normal.
2. **Sleeping:** Babies sleep a lot, usually 14-17 hours a day, but sleep patterns can be irregular.
3. **Crying:** It's normal for babies to cry, sometimes for up to

2-3 hours a day.

4. **Breathing:** Babies might breathe irregularly, especially when sleeping. Occasional pauses up to 10 seconds can be normal.

Common Signs Of Illness

1. A rectal temperature of 100.4°F (38°C) or higher in infants under 3 months should be evaluated by a doctor.
2. Persistent coughing, wheezing, or difficulty breathing.
3. Refusal to eat or drink for extended periods.
4. Persistent diarrhea or frequent vomiting can lead to dehydration.
5. Unusual or persistent rashes, especially if accompanied by fever.
6. Excessive irritability, lethargy, or unusual drowsiness.
7. Fewer wet diapers than usual, indicating possible dehydration.
8. Persistent diarrhea or constipation.

Signs Of Danger: When To Seek Immediate Medical Help

1. Rapid breathing, flaring nostrils, grunting, or blue lips.
2. Any fever in infants under 3 months or a high fever in older babies that doesn't reduce with medication.
3. Any seizure activity, even if it's brief.
4. Vomiting that continues for more than a few hours or is green/bloody.
5. Signs include dry mouth, no tears when crying, sunken eyes, and fewer than six wet diapers a day.
6. Extreme drowsiness, difficulty waking up, or not responding to stimuli.

7. Rash that spreads quickly, is accompanied by fever, or looks infected.
8. The soft spot on the top of the baby's head is bulging, indicating possible increased intracranial pressure.
9. Inconsolable crying for hours that can't be soothed.
10. Any head injury, fall, or accident that concerns you.

Monitoring Your Baby

- Keep a log of your baby's symptoms, including fever, feeding, diaper changes, and behavior changes.
- If something feels off, trust your instincts and consult your pediatrician.
- Attend all scheduled pediatric appointments for regular monitoring of your baby's health and development.

Understanding the difference between normal behaviors and signs of illness in your baby can be challenging. Regular monitoring, keeping an eye on changes in behavior, and maintaining open communication with your pediatrician are key strategies in ensuring your baby's health and well-being. Always err on the side of caution and seek medical advice if you have any concerns.

Deficiencies (Red Signs)

Deficiencies in newborns typically manifest as more subtle and gradual signs compared to the often acute and rapid onset of diseases.

While both deficiencies and diseases can impact a newborn's health, deficiencies tend to have a slower, progressive impact on growth and development, whereas diseases often prompt quicker and more urgent medical responses due to their immediate and severe symptoms. Recognizing these differences is crucial for timely intervention and treatment to ensure the newborn's health and well-being.

Iron Deficiency

Signs And Symptoms:

1. Look for paleness, especially in the face, inside the lips, and around the nails.
2. Unusual tiredness or low energy levels.
3. Refusal to eat or decreased interest in feeding.
4. Slower than expected growth and development.
5. Increased fussiness or irritability.
6. Increased susceptibility to infections.

When To Seek Help:

- If your baby exhibits several of these signs, consult your pediatrician for a blood test to check iron levels.

Vitamin D Deficiency

Signs And Symptoms:

1. Slower growth in height and weight.
2. Pain or tenderness in the bones, particularly the legs.
3. Delay in reaching milestones like sitting, crawling, or walking.
4. Weakness or floppiness in the muscles.
5. Increased frequency of colds or other respiratory infections.

When to Seek Help:

- If you notice these signs, especially if your baby is

exclusively breastfed without vitamin D supplementation, consult your pediatrician.

Calcium Deficiency

Signs And Symptoms:

1. Unusual twitching or cramping of muscles.
2. Teeth taking longer to emerge or appearing soft.
3. Increased fussiness or discomfort.
4. Lack of interest in feeding or eating.
5. Delayed physical growth and development.

When To Seek Help:

- If these symptoms are present, discuss with your pediatrician the possibility of calcium deficiency.

Vitamin B12 Deficiency

Signs And Symptoms:

1. Paleness or a slight yellowing of the skin and eyes.
2. Unusual tiredness and lethargy.
3. Delayed achievement of developmental milestones.
4. Reduced interest in feeding or eating.
5. Increased fussiness or crying.

When To Seek Help:

- Consult your pediatrician if you notice these symptoms, particularly if your baby is breastfed and the mother is vegan or vegetarian.

Iodine Deficiency

Signs And Symptoms:

1. Swelling in the neck due to an enlarged thyroid gland.

2. Slower physical and cognitive development.
3. Low energy levels and lethargy.
4. Sensitivity to cold temperatures.
5. Dry, flaky skin, and brittle hair.

When To Seek Help:

- If these signs are present, discuss with your pediatrician the need for iodine supplementation.

Zinc Deficiency

Signs And Symptoms:

1. Slower than expected growth in height and weight.
2. Reduced interest in feeding or eating.
3. Increased susceptibility to illnesses.
4. Slow healing of cuts and bruises.
5. Persistent rashes or skin lesions.

When To Seek Help:

- If your baby shows these symptoms, a pediatrician can recommend zinc supplementation.

Monitoring And Prevention

1. Regular Check-Ups: Ensure regular pediatric visits for growth and development monitoring.
2. Balanced Diet: Introduce a variety of foods appropriate for your baby's age to ensure balanced nutrition.
3. Breastfeeding and Supplementation: If breastfeeding, follow your pediatrician's advice on necessary supplements, especially vitamin D and iron.
4. Observe and Record: Keep track of your baby's eating habits, growth, and any changes in behavior or physical appearance.

When In Doubt

- Always seek medical advice if you suspect any deficiency or if your baby exhibits any of the warning signs mentioned.
- Adhere to your pediatrician's recommendations for dietary changes or supplements.

Nutritional deficiencies can have significant impacts on your baby's health and development. Being aware of the warning signs and seeking prompt medical advice can help ensure your baby receives the necessary nutrients for healthy growth and development.

Sources

1. Centers for Disease Control and Prevention. (2021). Iron Deficiency Anemia. Retrieved from CDC.
2. Mayo Clinic. (2021). Iron deficiency in children: Prevention tips for parents. Retrieved from Mayo Clinic.
3. American Academy of Pediatrics. (2019). Vitamin D: On the Double. Retrieved from HealthyChildren.org.
4. National Institutes of Health. (2020). Vitamin D. Retrieved from NIH.
5. KidsHealth. (2021). Calcium. Retrieved from KidsHealth.
6. National Institutes of Health. (2021). Calcium. Retrieved from NIH.
7. American Academy of Pediatrics. (2021). Vitamin B12 Deficiency. Retrieved from HealthyChildren.org.
8. National Institutes of Health. (2020). Vitamin B12. Retrieved from NIH.
9. World Health Organization. (2020). Iodine deficiency. Retrieved from WHO.

10. National Institutes of Health. (2021). Iodine. Retrieved from NIH.

11. National Institutes of Health. (2021). Zinc. Retrieved from NIH.

12. Mayo Clinic. (2021). Zinc supplements: What to know if you're thinking of adding one to your diet. Retrieved from Mayo Clinic.

Vaccines

What Are Vaccines And Why Are They Necessary For Newborns?

Vaccines are biological preparations that provide immunity to specific infectious diseases. They contain parts of a particular organism (antigen) that are either weakened or inactivated. These parts/antigens are injected/delivered into the body, triggering an immune response within the body. When vaccinated, the immune system recognizes the antigen as a threat and creates antibodies to fight it off. This process helps the body remember the pathogen, allowing it to respond quickly and effectively if exposed in the future. This process is much safer than the body learning to fight the actual pathogen because in this way the pathogen is much stronger and can easily overwhelm the immune system. It becomes even more dangerous in case of newborns because their immune systems are underdeveloped during this age.

Why are vaccines necessary for newborns?

Newborns have an underdeveloped immune system, making them more susceptible to infections. Vaccines help to protect them during this vulnerable period. Vaccines can prevent serious illnesses that can lead to severe complications or death, such as measles, polio, and whooping cough. Vaccinating children helps to establish herd immunity, protecting those who cannot be vaccinated, such as immunocompromised individuals. Preventing diseases through vaccination is far more cost-effective than treating them after they occur.

Common Views Against Vaccination

1. Some parents worry about potential side effects of vaccines, which are generally mild and temporary.
2. Misinformation about vaccines, often spread through social media and other channels, can lead to fear and reluctance.
3. Some parents refuse vaccines due to personal, religious, or philosophical beliefs.
4. Some believe that natural infection is better for developing immunity than vaccination.

So, are vaccines safe in my view?

Vaccines are a crucial tool for protecting the health of newborns and children. They are rigorously tested in clinical trials to ensure safety and efficacy, and after approval, their safety is continuously monitored through various surveillance systems. While vaccines can cause minor side effects like soreness at the injection site or mild fever, serious side effects are extremely rare. The benefits of vaccination, which include the prevention of life-threatening diseases and the promotion of herd immunity, far outweigh the potential risks. Misinformation and personal beliefs can cause fear, but it's important to rely on credible sources for accurate information. Natural immunity gained through infection can be dangerous, while vaccines offer a safer alternative.

Eradication Of Polio

Polio, a highly infectious viral disease, was eradicated in India due to a successful vaccination program. The polio vaccine campaign, known as the Pulse Polio Immunization Program, began in 1995. Through extensive efforts, including door-to-door immunization and nationwide awareness campaigns, India was declared polio-free in 2014 by the World Health Organization.

Vaccination Schedule

1st 6 Months Vaccine

Age	Vaccine
Birth to 15 Days	BCG
	OPV-0
6 weeks	OPV1+IPV1/OPV1
	DTwP1/DTaP1
	Hepatitis-B1
	Hib-1
	Pneumococcal Conjugate-1
	Rotavirus Vaccine-1
10 weeks	OPV2+IPV2/OPV2
	DTwP2/DTaP2
	Hepatitis-B2
	Hib-2
	Pneumococcal Conjugate-2
	Rotavirus Vaccine-2
14 weeks	OPV3+IPV3/OPV3
	DTwP3/DTaP3
	Hepatitis-B3

	Hib-3
	Pneumococcal Conjugate-3
	Rotavirus Vaccine-3

6 Months To 1 Year Vaccine

Age	Vaccine
6 Months	Flu Vaccine-1
7 Months	Flu Vaccine-2
9 Months	MMR1
10-12 Months	Typhoid Conjugate Vaccine
	Meningococcal Vaccine-1

1 To 2 Year Vaccine

Age	Vaccine
12 Months	Hepatitis A-1
	Japanese Encephalitis-1
13 Months	Japanese Encephalitis-2
	Meningococcal Vaccine-2
15 Months	MMR2
	Varicella-1
	Pneumococcal Booster
18 Months	OPV+IPV/OPV Booster
	DTwp+DTaP Booster
	Hib Booster
19 Months	Hepatitis A-2
2 Year	Varicella-2

After 2 Years Vaccine

Age	Vaccine
5 Years	DTwP/DTaP Booster+OPV
9-16 Years	Cervical Cancer Vaccine (HPV) (Only for Girls)
10 Years	Tdap/Td

16 Years	Tdap/Td
Every Year	Flu Vaccine

Diphtheria Pertussis & Tetanus (DPT) - Booster 2

The second of two doses of the DPT vaccine is recommended for children aged 5-6 years. It is administered via injection to protect against diphtheria, pertussis (whooping cough), and tetanus. Possible side effects include soreness, swelling at the injection site, fever, irritability, tiredness, loss of appetite, and vomiting.

10 YEARS Tetanus & Adult Diphtheria (Td)

This single-dose vaccine is administered via injection to protect against tetanus, which can result from contaminated wounds with Clostridium tetani spores. Diphtheria, a bacterial infection causing breathing difficulties, heart issues, paralysis, or death, is also prevented. Side effects may include pain, redness, swelling at the injection site, mild fever, headache, fatigue, and gastrointestinal symptoms.

16 YEARS Tetanus & Adult Diphtheria (Td)

Similarly, this single-dose vaccine is administered via injection to prevent tetanus and diphtheria. It protects against tetanus caused by Clostridium tetani spores and diphtheria, which can lead to severe respiratory problems, heart failure, paralysis, or fatality. Common side effects include pain, redness, swelling at the injection site, mild fever, headache, fatigue, and gastrointestinal symptoms.

Vaccines and Their Purposes

- **Bacillus Calmette-Guérin (BCG) Vaccine**
    - Protects against tuberculosis (TB).

- **Oral Polio Vaccine (OPV)**
  - Protects against poliovirus, which can cause paralysis.
- **Hepatitis B Birth Dose**
  - Protects against Hepatitis B, which attacks the liver.
- **Pentavalent - First Dose**
  - Provides immunity against Diphtheria, Pertussis (Whooping Cough), Tetanus, Hepatitis B, and Haemophilus influenzae type b (Hib).
- **Rotavirus Vaccine (RVV)**
  - Protects against rotaviruses, which cause severe diarrheal disease.
- **Pneumococcal Conjugate Vaccine (PCV) - First Dose**
  - Protects against meningitis, septicemia, pneumonia, sinusitis, and otitis media.
- **Measles Mumps & Rubella (MR) - First Dose**
  - Protects against measles, mumps and rubella.
- **Japanese Encephalitis (JE-1) - First Dose**
  - Protects against Japanese Encephalitis.
- **Diphtheria Pertussis & Tetanus (DPT) - Booster 1**
  - Protects against diphtheria, pertussis (whooping cough), and tetanus.

https://www.unicef.org/india/know-your-childs-immunization-schedule

https://www.ncbi.nlm.nih.gov/pmc/articles/PMC4928529/

Chapter 8

COMPLEXITIES OF PARENTING TODAY

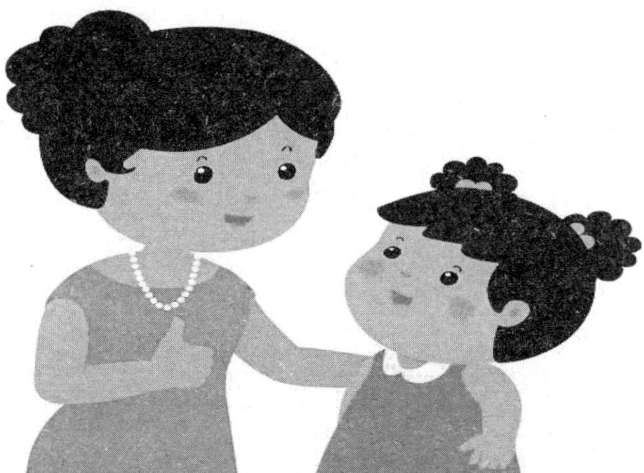

We talked about the culprit culture in the first chapter. A culture that makes parenting so complex and challenging, that parents have become clueless about the journeys that lay ahead. Right from psychological manipulation to nutrition, healthcare, upbringing, everything is jumbled. We can't trust the information that flows out there because layer by layer, our value chains have fallen down to corrupt capitalistic models. This is why it is important we know about the biggest complexities of parenting today. When you know that these exist and impact our thinking, you can make sound decisions by considering the factors that are affecting modern parenting.

Nutrition:

There is so much confusion regarding "the right food". What should you feed your child? Sugar or salt are they bad? Should dairy be allowed or not? See, I say that you can't even trust your "Ghar ka khaana" today. Once "ghar ka khaane" was the key for indian mothers to show their care and love towards their children. Just the phrase represented so many emotions for us Indians. The warmth of family, the love of our mothers, the care of our fathers and the nutrition packed in the simplicity of home cooked meals. But with the coming of modern practices no "khaana" is as healthy as it used to be.

The culprit is actually the ingredients, the modern food practices and the value chain through which we receive them. Our home cooked food comes mixed with unhealthy and refined oils, chemically prepared fruits and vegetables, packaged spices that use colors, additives and what not.

In the vast fields where our food grows, there are silent killers lurking beneath the surface. These are the chemicals and fertilizers we use on our crop yields to keep pests and weeds from harming our food crops. However, despite our efforts to confine their usage to the agricultural environment, the reality is that these substances find their way into the very foods we consume.

These chemicals find their way into the soil and water systems, entering the plants through roots or external contact. Once absorbed, these chemicals accumulate within the plant tissues, including the edible parts that we eventually consume. Additionally, some chemicals also persist in the soil or water sources, posing a risk of affecting subsequent crops or entering into groundwater supplies. “Hawa, paani, khaana sab polluted and compromised hai.”

Furthermore, during food processing, additional chemical treatments or preservatives are added to vegetables and fruits to bring out the color in them or to keep them fresher for a longer time. Even during transportation and storage, there is potential for further chemical exposure.

The concern therefore lies in the potential health effects of these chemical residues when ingested by humans.

When humans eat foods that have been treated with chemicals and fertilizers, these substances can end up inside our bodies.

Inside our bodies, these chemicals can cause problems. They might disrupt the way our hormones work, mess up how our bodies process food, or even harm our organs. That’s why it’s important to be careful about what you as a young mother eat and feed your child.

Malnutrition: A Public Health Crisis

Malnutrition – it actually means "bad nourishment" and includes all conditions that result from taking too little, too much, or an unbalance of nutrients. This is so far the single most high-profile breath-counting threat to global public health, according to the World Health Organisation (WHO), The consequence of malnutrition, both from undernutrition and overnutrition, is staggering in its contribution to the overall risk of disease and premature death.

Malnutrition comes in several forms, and there are a number of health problems that can result from it. Protein-energy malnutrition, a common issue seen among many developing nations which gives rise to multiple conditions such as Kwashiorkor and Marasmus etc. Stunting, severe wasting and weakened immunity, along with increased susceptibility to infections and resulting morbidities/mortalities, are some of the most extreme manifestations of undernutrition. Additionally vitamin and mineral deficiency also cause various diseases like anemia, scurvy rickets etc.

Alternatively, overnutrition which is more present in the developed world has a whole different set of challenges to cope with. If eating more than the optimal level of calories and an unhealthy displacement toward certain foods increases the risk of obesity, then obesity is a predecessor to diabetes, hypertension, cardiovascular diseases (CVD), kidney failure, liver issues such as cirrhosis and gallbladder issues. These are chronic conditions in most cases and can have a severe impact on the quality of living, is also something, which escalates the cost across all its expenditure structures.

Child Malnutrition In India

Malnutrition is a particularly alarming health problem in children of India. Just to remind you, 36% of children under five are stunted; 19 % are wasted, 32% are underweight and 3% overweight (National Institute of Nutrition). "These figures indicate that the problem of malnutrition, the double burden where undernutrition and overnutrition converge together. The extent of this problem can be judged by the Global Hunger Index score which is 28.7 and falls under the very serious category. "Underlying causes include a high level of economic disparity, where 74% of our population cannot afford an adequate diet and across South African, 39% is below the nutrient adequacy for activity," said Labadarios.

A Path To Resolution

To improve malnutrition, several aims should be taken into consideration, as mentioned earlier, including prevention and cure. The first one is a healthy diet that affects the ability to keep a healthy body. Community- based care programs can assist the public in making healthier eating decisions, such as increasing their fruit and vegetable intake and decreasing the amount of sugar and oils they have access to. Indeed, a solid healthcare system that includes immunization, detection and treatment of diseases and infections, oral rehydration, and routine deworming will assist in preventing malnutrition. Breast milk alone for the first half of a year of life, followed by continued breastfeeding during the first 15 to 18 months of life, is minimally required for children's nourishment and growth.

Prevention Strategies

Malnutrition can well be prevented by educating mothers

about food nutrition and hygiene, immunization and breast feeding along with weaning practices" (p. 67). Considering growth against a growth chart helps recognize children who are at risk of experiencing these deficiencies as soon as possible so that we may take control quickly. Targeting screening of high-risk groups along with good nutritional care and supplement feeding programs can reduce malnutrition to a considerable extent.

For example, wellness education in schools can raise awareness among children about good eating habits and exercise, which will result in leading a healthy life till their end of life. It's this kind of education that enables kids to grow up making better decisions so they can lead a healthier life and put an end to the vicious cycle of malnutrition.

All forms of malnutrition are serious public health issues with far-reaching effects. It will need a coordinated effort from people, communities, and governments to address this issue. We can effectively combat malnutrition by encouraging balanced diets, bolstering healthcare systems, and educating the public. By doing so, we can improve health outcomes and quality of life everywhere.

Post Covid Worries

Every time a little sniffle or cough appears, young moms can't help but worry. They question if their child is growing right, meeting weight goals, and doing everything perfectly.

When mothers come for a consultation to our hospital they often ask me questions about their child's growth, "how much should my child be gaining in a day doctor", and if I tell them that it should somewhere around 30 gms a day, some even go to the extent of buying weighing scales and weighing their child's growth everyday.

On top of that the constant flow of advice and the pressure to raise flawless kids only makes their stress worse. As our society grapples with the consequences of the culprit culture, the health landscape for children has become increasingly complex. There are various diseases and infections that are out there, ranging from common illnesses like colds and flu to more serious conditions such as pneumonia, ear infections, and gastrointestinal infections like gastroenteritis often caused by viruses, bacteria, or other pathogens that can easily spread in daycare settings, schools, or other communal environments where children interact closely. Then there are lifestyle related illnesses like the rising rates of obesity, diabetes, mental health disorders, and other health problems that present significant challenges for parents, particularly young mothers who often find themselves overwhelmed and anxious about their children's well-being.

Moreover, post-COVID, mothers have become even more conscious about their child's health and well-being. The pandemic has heightened awareness about the importance of hygiene, vaccinations, and overall health practices. While this increased vigilance may bring added worries, it also empowers mothers to take proactive steps in keeping their children safe and healthy.

In navigating through these anxieties, it's essential for young mothers to seek support from healthcare providers, family members, and other trusted sources. Seek reliable information from trusted sources. Even in this book, I will try my best to talk more about the illnesses that children mostly encounter in the later chapters.

The Age Of Misinformation

In today's digital age, social media has become an integral part of our lives, offering unprecedented connectivity, information and convenience. Millions of parents reach out to me through social media, in fact I have been called "The viral doctor" at times because of the magnanimity of social following people have poured into my accounts with. However, within the framework of the "culprit culture," social media presents a double-edged sword, with both benefits and pitfalls for children and families.

Social media platforms are designed to be captivating, offering a constant stream of content tailored to individual preferences and interests. I would say for babies, it is harmful in every sense and parents should not engage their infants, toddlers in it. For children, the colorful visuals, interactive features, and endless possibilities for entertainment can be incredibly enticing. From engaging games and videos to virtual communities and instant messaging, social media offers a virtual playground where children can explore, connect, and express themselves.

Despite its allure, we all know that excessive use of social media has detrimental effects on children's development and well-being. However, social media is harmful in certain aspects for parents as well.

Social media often presents a highlight reel of other parents' lives, showcasing their seemingly perfect moments and achievements. This can create a sense of pressure to measure up and portray our own lives in a similar light. However, constantly comparing ourselves to others can lead to feelings of inadequacy and self-doubt, impacting our confidence as parents.

Excessive use of social media can detract from quality time spent with our children. When we're constantly checking our phones or scrolling through social media feeds, we may miss out on valuable moments and opportunities for meaningful connection with our children. This can weaken the parent-child bond and hinder effective communication and emotional support.

Social media can also exacerbate parental anxiety, fueling worries about our children's well-being and comparing our parenting choices to others. I often see young mothers spending their entire time, learning new things about their babies from social media content. This overload of information creates more harm than good. It increases feelings of stress and guilt.

I would say rather than engaging in social media, you and your child should both spend time in knowing and experiencing life. I will again remind you of the same thing, "nature is kind". You, your child, your body, they all have their roles to perform, and you will get the hang of it. And wherever you think you need help, seek it from people who care about you and your child's welfare. Seek help from your family, from your doctor, your friends but don't blindly trust everything you see on social media. And don't fall into the pit of comparison. No person who started doing something new, became perfect at it all at once. Take baby steps along with your child, and you will understand everything.

Most importantly recognize that social media often presents a skewed version of reality and to prioritize self-care and mental health.

Babies Need Humans, Not Screens- UNICEF

The world out there is constantly fighting for your attention and most importantly your money. The capitalistic world out there wants to put you into a loop of wanting the products and services that are not at all necessary for your life or your children's.

As this wanting is what creates the cycle of profits for them.

Today's culture has fostered an environment where addiction, be it to digital devices, substances, or unhealthy foods, has become rampant. These addictions distract our children, impairing their ability to focus and learn, while also posing serious long-term health risks.

On an everyday basis, I come across parents who distract their children with phones. A little tantrum and the child is handed a mobile phone. A child who is crying on top of his lungs, gives him a phone and he forgets everything, enjoying the addiction of scrolling and just watching. Appealing and bright colors, sounds, new people, it keeps them engaged for sure but little by little their brain is learning addiction.

During the early years, a child's brain undergoes rapid growth, forming neural connections at an astonishing rate. These connections are strengthened by interacting with the environment through sensory experiences, motor activities, and social interactions. However, too much screen time can limit these crucial interactions, slowing down cognitive development and affecting skills such as language, problem-solving, and critical thinking.

Patricia Kuhl is one of the world's leading brain scientists.

She runs experiments with more than 4,000 babies each year. "What we've discovered is that little babies, under a year old, do not learn from a machine," based on several brain scans she has conducted during her research. "Even if you show them captivating videos, the difference in learning is extraordinary. You get genius learning from a live human being, and you get zero learning from a machine."

So all those songs on certain Youtube channels, all those poems being played on music systems, research says children learn better from humans and not from machines.

Perhaps that is why the World Health Organization recommends no screen time for babies under 2 and no more than one hour of screen time a day for those aged 2 to 4.

Language development relies heavily on verbal interaction and engagement with caregivers. Screens can reduce the time children spend in active, two-way communication, leading to delays in language acquisition and poorer verbal skills. The brain misses out on the rich linguistic input needed for robust language development, hindering their ability to communicate effectively.

Attention and focus are also impacted by screen time. Young children naturally have short attention spans, and their ability to focus is still developing. The rapid, ever-changing images on screens can train the brain to expect constant stimulation, making it harder for children to concentrate on tasks that require sustained attention. This can potentially lead to attention disorders like ADHD.

Young children need their dose of boredom. It teaches them how to cope with frustration and control their impulses. If they are constantly being stimulated by screens, they forget how to rely on themselves or others for entertainment. This leads to frustration and hinders imagination and motivation. Physical development is another critical area affected by screen time. Physical activity is essential for developing fine and gross motor skills, coordination, and overall physical health. Time spent on screens often replaces time that could be spent on physical play and exploration, resulting in weaker muscle development, poor coordination, and an increased risk of obesity and related health issues.

Sleep patterns are crucial for brain development, memory consolidation, and overall health. The blue light emitted by screens can interfere with melatonin production, a hormone that regulates sleep. It can lead to difficulties falling asleep, disrupted sleep patterns, and insufficient sleep, all of which are essential for healthy brain and body development.

Lastly, social and emotional skills in children develop through direct interaction with caregivers and peers. Screens replace these face-to-face interactions, reducing opportunities for children to learn and practice social cues, empathy, and emotional regulation. This can lead to difficulties in forming healthy relationships and managing emotions. Research has shown that screen time inhibits young children's ability to read faces and learn social skills, two key factors needed to develop empathy. Face-to-face interactions are the only way young children learn to understand non-verbal cues and interpret them. Exposure to screens reduces babies' ability to read human emotion and control their frustration.

Signs Of Phone Addiction To Look For In Infants And Toddlers:

1. **Constant Distraction:** If you find yourself frequently handing your phone to your child to distract them whenever they become fussy or restless, it could be a sign of reliance on screen time for soothing.
2. **Resistance To Transition:** Notice if your child throws tantrums or becomes upset when you take the phone away or switch off the screen. This resistance to transitioning away from screens may indicate dependence or addiction.
3. **Excessive Screen Time:** Pay attention to the amount of time your child spends in front of screens each day. If it exceeds the recommended guidelines for their age group and interferes with other activities like playtime or social interaction, it may be cause for concern.
4. **Withdrawal Symptoms:** Watch for signs of withdrawal when screen time is limited or removed. These could include increased irritability, restlessness, or difficulty settling down for sleep.
5. **Lack Of Interest In Other Activities:** Notice if your child shows little interest in engaging with toys, books, or outdoor play when screens are not available. This may indicate that screens have become their primary source of entertainment and stimulation.
6. **Physical Symptoms:** Be mindful of any physical symptoms that may arise from excessive screen time, such as strained eyes, headaches, or poor posture. These can be indicators of prolonged screen use.

- Between 18 and 24 months screen time should be limited to watching educational programming with a caregiver.
- For children 2-5, limit non-educational screen time to about 1 hour per weekday and 3 hours on the weekend days.
- For ages 6 and older, encourage healthy habits and limit activities that include screens.

So where does this leave us?

In today's digital age, information is indeed akin to currency, and just like managing finances, it's essential to be discerning about where you invest your trust. Much like avoiding bad debt, seeking information from reputable and credible sources ensures you're making wise investments in knowledge.

Childcare is both inherent and ascribed meaning it is both in you and can be learnt by you. The reason behind writing this book is, I, as a doctor, do not just focus on the biological and physiological aspect of childcare, rather I believe that comprehensive care from all systems involved in the process are necessary to raise a better future for our country, our families and our homes. When you bear a child, the child is not just yours; in your arms resides the future of this nation, this society, your community and if we invest in equipping parents with the science backed knowledge of childcare I think we can create wonderful generations that can not only survive the culprit culture but also build one that is sustainable and better for all of us.

Being a parent is not a personal affair, it's a responsibility on me as a doctor, on you as parents, on society as the teacher and on the country as the provider. So, learn about how you can play your part best because knowledge and information is the biggest currency today.

Learning about how to be a good parent is super important. Learn to understand your child better and know what to do in different situations. Just take this small example, you think by vaccinating your child, you are only helping your child prevent those diseases but if you look at the bigger picture, your contribution towards vaccination programmes is boosting the health care in the country. It is helping the government to eradicate these diseases from our land and territory.

And when parents know about things they can take better care of their children.

In our journey through the challenges of modern parenting, let's hold tight to the incredible bond between a parent, a child and the doctor. From day one, our kids rely on us for love, guidance, and safety. It's our job to shield them from the not-so-great stuff out there until they're old enough to handle it themselves.

Until our kids grow up a bit, it's up to us to be their protectors. We can shape their world, teach them right from wrong, and help them stay strong when things get tough. By spending quality time together and being there for them, we're giving them a strong base to stand on.

Sure, there's a lot of tricky stuff out there like social media and junk food ads, but as parents, we've got a superpower: love. By talking openly, setting rules, and being good role models, we can help our kids deal with the ups and downs of the new world.

Chapter 9

3D'S: DUA, DAWA AND DOCTOR

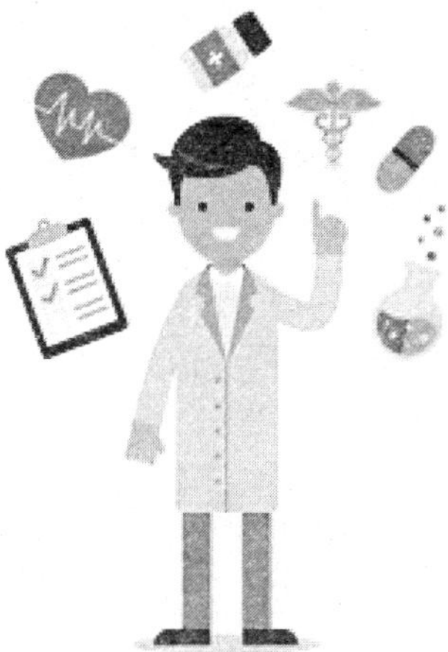

As parents, the fear of losing your child to an illness often tops the list of anxieties. It is a fear that can be paralyzing, making every sniffle and fever feel like a looming catastrophe. There are sometimes smaller complications that can be dealt with little medical intervention but sometimes complications take bigger magnitudes. And for times like these, I want to tell you that nothing is stronger than faith and belief.

I want to provide you with a perspective–one grounded in hope, resilience, and the extraordinary power of human will. Through the lens of some of the most challenging cases I have encountered in my career, I want to convey this message that even in the face of the direst circumstances, there is always a glimmer of hope.

In these stories, you will see the incredible strength and tenacity that children possess, the unwavering dedication of medical professionals, and the profound impact of a supportive and loving environment. Each case is a testament to the idea that when we combine dua (prayer), dawa (medicine), and the tireless efforts of a dedicated doctor, we can overcome even the most formidable obstacles.

In the following pages, I will share stories that highlight these intersections. These are not just tales of medical triumphs but narratives that underscore the importance of hope and the human spirit. They serve as reminders that no matter how daunting a situation may appear, there is always room for miracles when faith, medicine, and human determination come together.

As you read these stories, I hope they bring you comfort and reassurance. Remember that you are not alone in your fears and anxieties. Every parent worries, and every doctor understands the weight of these concerns. Together, with dua, dawa, and the steadfast support of a dedicated medical team, we can navigate through the darkest times and find the light of hope.

The Importance Of Courage In Medicine

To survive as a doctor, you need courage. Courage to stand amidst wailing patients and gather the last ounces of strength to alleviate their pain or save their lives. While the mere sight of blood may be mortifying for some, a doctor often sees the entire physiology cut into pieces and then stitches the pieces back together, allowing the human on the table to live again.

It's a conundrum: to live again, a patient must first let go at the doctor's table. A doctor's journey is made through their patients' stories. The quiet corridors of the hospital can change in a second into the turbulence of a medical emergency. Amidst beeping monitors and hurried footsteps, a doctor rushes to rescue lives, leaving behind rest and personal time to fulfill their duty.

The Doctor-Patient Connection

What is it that renders the tag of "Bhagwan" or "God" to a doctor? Perhaps it is the profound connection forged with each patient, where their very existence hangs in the balance of the healer's hands. The power to decide life and death, to navigate the delicate dance between hope and despair, rests solely upon the shoulders of those who wear the white coat.

The pressure of becoming a doctor is immense. It intersects with every aspect of your life, to the point that you lose all parts of yourself to become one with the identity of a doctor. We have to be there with people during their most vulnerable and dreaded times. Death, loss, and grief become daily sights, making it easy to lose oneself to the sadness of our existence.

People often ask me, “How is it that you appear to be so happy and energetic all the time? What makes little babies forget about their pain during vaccinations? What keeps you going?” My experience and exposure to life’s nature taught me a different aspect of being a doctor. When a person, couple, or family comes to me, they come with the hope of being free of their problems. They consult me for solutions. Sometimes, we know the inevitable morbidity of certain cases, but I try my best not to give up before God takes matters into his own hands.

Human Will And Resilience

I have seen the worst cases, where the hope of a child’s survival was almost non-existent. However, I have also witnessed the power of human will and resilience during these times. Some children have defeated death where there was no hope. I always say, “Dua, dawa and Doctor should always work together.” When you encounter these incidents, which sometimes appear closer to miracles, you start appreciating life and its ways. This allows me to connect with the people who come to my hospital searching for a cure and respite.

The Power Of Empathy

Numerous studies highlight the positive impact of a doctor’s behavior and connection on patients. One notable study is “The Empathy Effect: How Physician Empathy Affects Patient Outcomes,” published in Academic Medicine in 2017. This study delves into the intricate dynamics of doctor-patient interactions, shedding light on the pivotal role of empathy in shaping clinical outcomes.

The study's findings reveal a cascade of positive effects stemming from empathetic physician-patient interactions. Improved patient satisfaction emerges as a cornerstone of this paradigm, as patients feel valued and respected when their doctors demonstrate empathy. Moreover, empathy significantly influences treatment adherence, as patients are more likely to follow prescribed treatment plans when they feel understood and supported by their physicians.

The Amazing Human Will

As I reflect on my journey as a doctor, there are a few cases that can never leave my memory. These children who were brought to me were in critical stages, and each one had their own story to tell.

These cases are a reminder that nothing beats human will and resilience and no matter whatever situation you are in, if you have the resolve to get out of it and make your life better, trust me Universe or should I say Science will offer you a solution and guide you to it.

One case that stands out vividly was the case of an eleven-year-old girl, her life was hanging in the balance as she battled against, Atypical pneumonia, pulmonary hemorrhage, and multiple organ failure. Atypical pneumonia, unlike the typical bacterial or viral pneumonia, often presents with more severe symptoms and can be challenging to treat. Pulmonary hemorrhage, characterized by bleeding in the lungs, further compounded her condition, leading to respiratory distress and organ dysfunction.

We immediately initiated intensive care measures, including mechanical ventilation to support her breathing and medications to stabilize her condition. What followed was days of medical intervention, I would sit by her side waiting for her condition to stabilize. For this child me and my team forgot all the segregations of duty, and we worked tirelessly to somehow get her out of the critical condition. Days turned into nights, each moment fraught with uncertainty as we watched over her, willing her to pull through.

Then, after eight agonizing days, of her being into a coma, a glimmer of hope emerged—she opened her eyes. It was a moment of triumph, a testament to the unwavering dedication of everyone involved in her care. Slowly but surely, she shifted from the ventilator to oxygen support and in a month's time she began to regain her strength.

When the time finally came for her to leave the hospital, it was a moment of profound joy and gratitude. We watched her walk back on her two feet and that was what made every ounce of our effort worth it.

A few days later I even received a call from her family, overwhelmed with emotions, telling me that they had made a pilgrimage to Haji Ali to pray for my wellness and to offer their thanks—a gesture that touched me deeply and served as a reminder of the power of compassion and resilience.

Premature Baby

Another case that is imprinted in my memory is of a little baby girl. It was a typical day in the hospital when the mother of a newborn baby girl, barely clinging to life, arrived at our doorstep.

The baby, born prematurely at just six months and weighing a mere 600 grams, was facing a battle for survival from the moment she entered this world. Premature birth, particularly when accompanied by low birth weight, poses a multitude of challenges and potential complications due to the underdeveloped organs and immature bodily systems of the infant. One of the primary complications associated with premature birth is Respiratory Distress Syndrome (RDS). Premature infants often lack sufficient surfactant–a substance in the lungs that helps keep air sacs open. Without enough surfactant, the air sacs collapse, making breathing difficult and leading to respiratory distress syndrome.

Another significant complication is Intraventricular Hemorrhage (IVH). The blood vessels in the brains of premature babies are delicate and prone to bleeding. IVH occurs when these blood vessels rupture, resulting in bleeding in the ventricles of the brain. This can lead to neurological complications and long-term developmental issues.

Necrotizing Enterocolitis (NEC) is a severe gastrointestinal condition that predominantly affects premature infants. It involves inflammation and damage to the intestinal tissue, which can progress to tissue death (necrosis), perforation of the bowel, and life-threatening infections.

Premature infants are also more susceptible to infections due to their underdeveloped immune systems. These infections, which can include sepsis, pneumonia, and meningitis, require prompt treatment with antibiotics and careful monitoring.

Additionally, premature babies may struggle to regulate their body temperature due to limited fat stores, making them vulnerable to hypothermia. Maintaining a warm environment is crucial for their well-being.

Feeding difficulties are common among premature infants, as they may have underdeveloped sucking and swallowing reflexes. Specialized feeding techniques or tube feeding may be necessary to ensure adequate nutrition and growth.

Furthermore, premature birth and low birth weight can impact a baby's growth and development, leading to delays in physical, cognitive, and emotional development. Early intervention and multidisciplinary care are essential to minimize these effects and promote optimal outcomes for these vulnerable newborns.

So, vulnerable to everything mentioned above, this child was extremely underweight and in addition to that had a premature birth.

We immediately initiated treatment, placing the baby on a ventilator to support her fragile respiratory system. Over the ensuing weeks, she remained under intensive care, her condition fluctuating between hope and despair. It was a challenging time, filled with uncertainty and apprehension as we fought to save her life.

But as the days turned into months, we began to see signs of progress. Despite the odds stacked against her, the baby's condition gradually stabilized, her tiny body growing stronger with each passing day. It was a testament to the dedication of our medical team and the resilience of the human spirit.

Eventually, the baby was able to leave the hospital, her health greatly improved from when she first arrived. Her mother, overwhelmed with gratitude, tied a rakhi around my wrist—a symbol of the bond forged between us through the shared experience of her daughter's journey to recovery.

The Wrong Diagnosis

As I sit down to recall one of the most challenging cases I've encountered in my career, the memory of a young child's struggle remains stuck to me.

I was at the hospital when I received a call from a frantic relative—a child was in critical condition, his face grotesquely swollen, and his family was desperate for answers. The person on the phone told me that a few days back the child was rushed to the nearest hospital where a diagnosis was given that the child was ingested with acid which had caused this reaction. He requested if I could examine the case and help them out, I asked them if they could take the chances, to bring the child to our hospital

Upon their arrival at the hospital, I witnessed a distressing scene—the child, barely a few years old, writhing in pain, his parents standing beside him in worry. With a quick assessment, it became apparent that something was seriously wrong. His face was swollen beyond recognition, and his labored breathing hinted at underlying complications. I suspected it was not an acid ingestion rather a case of diptheria.

I quickly ordered a test for the infection and after conducting a series of diagnostic tests, the grim reality set in—the rare bacterial infection known as diphtheria had indeed taken hold of the child's fragile body, wreaking havoc on his respiratory system and threatening his life. Diphtheria is a bacterial infection caused by Corynebacterium diphtheriae. It primarily affects the mucous membranes of the throat and nose, leading to the formation of a thick, gray coating in the throat that can obstruct breathing and swallowing.

The bacteria release toxins that can cause damage to various organs in the body, leading to serious complications such as heart failure, paralysis, and even death if left untreated.

Diphtheria is highly contagious and spreads through respiratory droplets from coughing or sneezing. It can also be transmitted by coming into contact with objects or surfaces contaminated with the bacteria.

The gravity of the situation weighed heavily on me as I grappled with the enormity of the task ahead. In addition to this the child's father was a truck driver who could not afford his treatment, that too in the private facilities.

However, there are certain situations where the life and situation takes precedence over money and gains. And this was one, so we offered to treat the child for free, however, his father did cover a portion of the charges.

For days on end, we fought tirelessly to save the child's life, his condition teetering on the brink of collapse. Prolonged exposure of 17 days to the ventilator had left his lungs scarred, and his body weakened, but we refused to give up hope. Round-the-clock care became our mantra as we navigated intensive care and fragility of the situation.

Slowly but surely, the child began to show signs of improvement—a flicker of hope amidst the darkness of despair. With each passing day, his condition stabilized, his body responding to the treatment with remarkable resilience.

Weeks turned into months as we continued to monitor his progress, never losing sight of the ultimate goal—to see him walk out of the hospital healthy and whole. And when the day finally arrived for him to leave our care, it was with a sense of profound gratitude that we bid him farewell, knowing that against all odds, we, his family and him all had emerged victorious.

This particular case is a testimony to how important diagnosis is in the treatment process. Diagnosis is the cornerstone of effective treatment. Without identifying the correct underlying issue, any treatment administered can be not only ineffective but also potentially harmful. This principle has been a guiding force throughout my career, shaping how I approach every patient and case.

I've often found myself playing the role of a detective. Unlike a typical detective who solves crimes, my mission is to solve medical mysteries. Every patient is like a puzzle, with symptoms serving as the pieces. Some cases are straightforward, with all the pieces fitting together neatly. However, more often than not, especially in pediatrics, the pieces are scattered and unclear. Children may not be able to describe their symptoms accurately, and parents might provide fragmented information based on their observations. It's my job to piece together these clues to form a coherent picture of what's wrong.

A good detective listens more than they speak. Similarly, in medicine, listening to the patient and their family is crucial. Parents often notice subtle changes in their children's behavior and health that might seem insignificant but can be critical in diagnosing a condition. Observing a child's behavior, interactions, and physical responses during the examination can also provide vital clues. Like detectives, doctors must ask the right questions to uncover hidden details. This involves not only understanding the current symptoms but also delving into the patient's medical history, family history, and lifestyle. Each question is designed to gather more information, helping to narrow down potential diagnoses. In pediatrics, this means engaging with both the child and the parents, ensuring that even the smallest detail isn't overlooked.

Looking back on the challenging time I faced with this case, I am reminded how in the face of adversity, humans find strength; in moments of uncertainty, we discover hope and how when your intention is pure, results show up as miracles. And as the child took his first tentative steps towards recovery, I knew that our efforts had not been in vain–that sometimes, miracles do happen when you least expect them. It is often said that with the right intention and the favorability of time come together, "acchi neeyat' the right intention can even dig a hole into the sky.

Intersection

In my journey as a doctor, there's one particular case etched deeply in my memory, reminding me of the complexities that often accompany the practice of medicine. It revolves around a child born into a family where marriages between close relatives are customary, a practice prevalent in certain religious communities. This cultural norm, while deeply ingrained, can sometimes lead to the manifestation of congenital deformities and genetic disorders in newborns. The mother who sought my help had already experienced the devastating loss of a two-month-old baby due to similar health issues, intensifying the gravity of the situation.

Upon examining the child, it became evident that his condition was indeed the result of a genetic disorder.

I learnt that she was married to a close relative in her family, who had left her as he was an addict, she was staying with her mother with meager resources to sustain themselves.

And in addition to this her child is struggling with a genetic disorder that is going to require heavy treatments.

In this particular case, I saw the intersection of so many problems in our society, the cultural practices, the social evils and the medical problems, all largely at play. We changed our approach to deal with this case, caring for both the mother and the child, sidelining the financial constraints of the family and just focusing on the caregiving aspect.

This is a recent case, so his diagnosis is still under progress but I hope that we can all learn a few more lessons with this case, going beyond just the medical intervention and offering comprehensive care.

The Instinct

In my career as a doctor, there's a case that stands out as a testament to the power of doctor's instincts and the willingness to take risks in the face of adversity. It revolves around a young child affectionately known as Duggu, whose life was threatened by a rare and severe condition.

Eight months ago, Duggu's world was turned upside down when his brain became inflamed, giving rise to pockets of pus that wreaked havoc within his fragile skull. His condition was dire, his brain shrinking under the relentless assault of infection, with each passing day bringing his condition closer to a disaster waiting to happen.

As a doctor, I was confronted with a daunting challenge, one that tested not only my medical expertise but also my resolve and conviction. Neurosurgeons were wary of the risks involved, they hesitated to intervene, fearing the potential for catastrophic bleeding that could endanger the life of a young child or at the least impair his brain development.

In the midst of uncertainty, my instincts guided me to take action, defying the norms of conventional wisdom. With determination, my team embraced the responsibility, assuring the family that their kid was gonna be fine.

Duggu's procedure involved extracting the puss out of the brain, and it was high risk surgery. My team went in with the resolve to save his life in any way possible. And it turned out to be like that. Duggu fought valiantly against the odds, his tiny body battling against the relentless onslaught of disease and the complexity of procedure. Through the procedures and treatments, he endured, and we endured despite the immense challenges that his condition presented.

The pockets of pus receded, the inflammation subsided, and his brain began to heal.

Eight months later, Duggu is happy and healthy, more so, his brain development is completely normal, casting aside any doubts I had of impairment. His case is a powerful example of perseverance and the triumph of the human spirit. Duggu's journey serves as a reminder that sometimes, the greatest victories are born from the depths of adversity.

As we reach the end of this chapter, I hope the stories shared have provided you with a sense of hope and reassurance. The journey of parenthood is filled with moments of joy, but it also comes with its share of fears and anxieties, especially when it comes to your child's health. Through the experiences recounted here, it is clear that even in the face of seemingly insurmountable challenges, there is always a way forward.

Chapter 10

PARENTING AND UNDERSTANDING YOUR CHILD

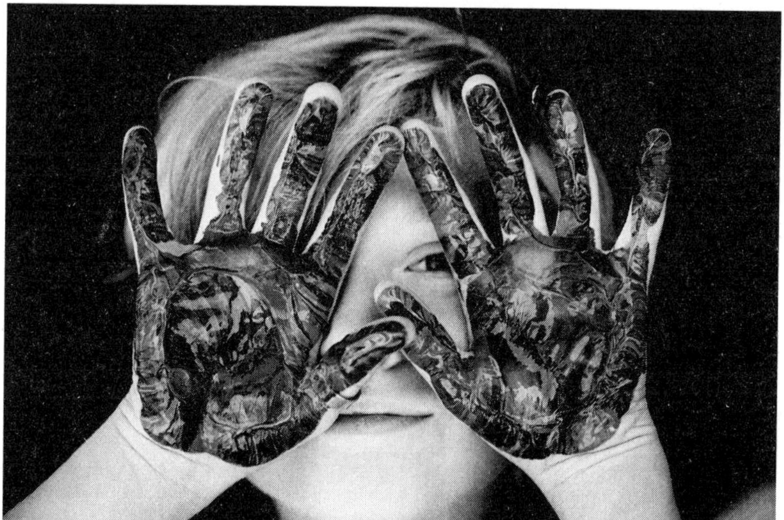

Raising a child is the most difficult and most grown-up thing I have ever had to do. It acts as a watershed between adulthood and childhood. On one hand, you break away from your childlike nature, and on the other, you become childlike. This duality is both beautiful and challenging, marking a profound shift in your identity and responsibilities.

Being a parent is daunting and confusing, and it carries a weighty responsibility. I understand this deeply because I, too, am a father of two boys. I know how overwhelming this journey can be, and for mothers, it is even more so, as your body, mind, and psyche undergo significant changes. The transformation is holistic, affecting every facet of your being. However, despite the difficult parts, a child gives you a fresh start in life. They offer you a chance to correct everything that went wrong in your life and set the record straight for the life coming ahead. A child is a new beginning, a chance to nurture and guide a life from scratch, learning and growing alongside them.

With this understanding, it is crucial for a parent to acknowledge that each child is unique. And one solution doesn't fit all. We try to fit whatever we have learnt of an "ideal child" on everyone. We tend to force our own set of ideas on these young children who don't even know the world yet. Just know that, your child is seeing the world through your eyes and whatever you are showing them, they will keep it safe for the rest of their life.

Often, as adults, we tend not to take children seriously. We consider their advice, stories, and interests to be of less importance than ours, and sometimes the pressures of life overshadow our bond with them. This is what creates a gap between us and our children, a gap that can be difficult to bridge if not addressed early on. Always remember that children are their own persons and they deserve respect too. They have their dignity, and as parents, we should know how to teach them valuable lessons without disrespecting or indignifying them. While they are under our care, they are individuals as well, with their thoughts, feelings, and aspirations.

Listening actively to your children is paramount. Value their opinions and encourage them to express their feelings and thoughts without fear of being dismissed or ridiculed. Empower their decision-making by offering choices and respecting their decisions, even if they are not perfect. Provide a safe space at home where they feel loved and free to be themselves. Encourage openness, making it clear they can come to you with any problem without fear of judgment.

Model respectful behavior by treating them and others with respect. Acknowledge your own mistakes and apologize, showing them that owning up to one's mistakes is a strength. Balance guidance with freedom by offering support without being overly controlling, allowing them to explore and learn from their experiences. Celebrate their achievements, no matter how small, and encourage them to pursue their interests and passions. Promote their self-esteem and confidence through positive reinforcement and by encouraging their self-expression in various forms.

Secondly There are anxieties around raising "perfect and high-achieving children." It's natural to want the best for your children, to dream of their success, and to envision a bright future filled with accomplishments. However, the relentless pursuit of perfection can place an undue burden on your child, leading to stress, anxiety, and a potential loss of self-identity.

It's essential to understand that pressuring children to excel in areas they are not passionate about can have adverse effects. Instead of thriving, they might feel overwhelmed and resentful. The constant push to meet unrealistic expectations can stifle their creativity, diminish their self-esteem, and foster a fear of failure. As parents, our role should not be to mold our children into our vision of perfection but to support and guide them as they discover their own paths.

Encourage your children to explore their interests and passions. Help them understand the importance of commitment and hard work in achieving their goals, but also emphasize the joy of learning and growing. Support them in their endeavors and celebrate their efforts, regardless of the outcome. This approach fosters a love for learning and a willingness to take on challenges without the paralyzing fear of falling short of perfection.

Ultimately, the goal of parenting is not to create "perfect" children but to raise well-rounded, compassionate, and confident individuals who are capable of navigating life's challenges with grace and resilience.